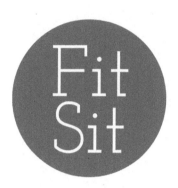

BACK FOR THE FUTURE

The Baby Boomer's Age-Busting Guide
to Better Movement

Stewart Hamblin

CONTENTS

Acknowledgments ·vii

Introduction · ix

1 / Side-bending—the key to balance · · · · · · · · · · · · · · · · · 15

2 / Reaching: how to use the spine to support the arms · · · · · · 55

3 / Flexion and extension · 89

4 / Feet, knees, and hips · 123

5 / Circles · 143

6 / Coming to stand effortlessly · 161

7 / Standing and walking from your centre · · · · · · · · · · · · · · 203

8 / Negotiating stairs with confidence · · · · · · · · · · · · · · · · · 235

9 / Conclusion · 261

Resources · 271

About the author · 273

ACKNOWLEDGMENTS

Following the publication of my first book during the COVID lockdown, I have become known as something of a specialist for my chair-based work. The origins of the material set out in this book started with one of my very first students, the late and much-loved Deidre Goodman (1927-2017). Deidre's daughter, Diffy, had asked me if I could help her mother with her movement, and I worked with Deidre regularly on Monday mornings until shortly before her death. That hour, in Deidre's company, was one of the highlights of my week. We often had a good gossip; one of the reasons I love my work is that it's so very social.

Despite being in a lot of pain from a crumbling spine, Deidre was such fun to be with, and I was humbled by her determination to improve the way that she could move. Out of necessity, the only safe place to work with Deidre was in a chair. The challenge for me as a teacher was to devise safe ways of working with her that would help her, challenge her appropriately, and engage her lively curiosity. She always wanted to know why we were doing something and what good it would do her. The fact that she had forgotten most of it by the next week was neither here nor there. It was with Deidre that I first began to explore using a stick as a teaching prop to tease movement out of her spine. Wherever you are in heaven, Deidre, thank you for being the inspiration for what was to come. I think you would be rather pleased with how that work has developed.

I have discovered that I love writing books and the opportunity writing gives me to share the work that I do. I have, however, also discovered that writing a book is a joint endeavour, and I need to thank more than a few people for their help.

To my past teachers, Lesley Ackland, Garet Newell, Jeremy Krauss, and Michelle Turner—thank you, once again, for having been so generous with your knowledge.

To Mrs Ann Kanter: thank you for allowing me to use your beautiful studio at Wardley to take the photographs and for all your support of my teaching over the years. It has been such fun and a privilege to work with you and your family.

Thank you to Phil and Joanna Jesson for your wise mentoring and for the title suggestion. It's brilliant, Phil.

Thank you to Mark, Sarah, and Denise of D. Norton & Son Ironmongers, Uppingham, for all the sticks. You guys are the best.

Thank you to my mum, of course, and an extra dollop of thanks to my big sister, Liz, for all the photographs, cups of tea, and company. Along with all my family, you have both been truly awesome.

I have the best students (adults and children) in the world! I would like to name and thank you all individually, but space does not permit. I thank you for being my true teachers, for allowing me to experiment, for being open to trying something new, for coming to class and workshops, for putting up with my long absences while I worked on other projects, for supporting me through family bereavements, and most of all for your friendship. This book would not have been possible without you. I thank you from the bottom of my heart.

Any and all errors are, of course, entirely mine.

INTRODUCTION

'Baby Boomers' *or* 'Boomers *—the generation often defined as people born from 1946-1964 during the mid-20th century baby boom (Wikipedia).*

"You are only as young as your spine is flexible" —JOSEPH PILATES

How well you age has everything to do with how well you move.

How well you move, in turn, has everything to do with your ability to use your core.

As people get older, they tend not to move from their core. It's a bad habit that they have developed that has very little to do with their age. It's as if their middle—their spine and pelvis—has become a black hole absorbing movement as opposed to transmitting it.

Over time this habit can lead to painful joints, poor balance, stiff necks, bad backs, breathing difficulties, and a host of other movement-related problems that begin to erode a person's quality of life, sense of wellbeing, and independence. I see it happening to Baby Boomers all around me.

The good news is that it's quite easy, whatever your age, to change this movement habit, using a simple but effective technique that will re-activate some fundamental movement skills which you mastered when you were much younger, and which—crazy as it may sound—you have probably forgotten that you could do. Let me explain briefly.

Every neurotypical child, as they pass through their developmental milestones, discovers through trial and error that their spine and pelvis are, in effect, an amazing suspension system that can support their movement and balance.

Toddlers learn how to side-bend, twist, rotate, flex, and extend their spines in such a way that will support the movement of their head so that they can get on with the busy job of exploring the world and having fun.

We tend to take these acquired movement skills so much for granted that we don't notice, over time, that if we fail to use them, bad things begin to happen to our movement, joints, and balance.

There are lots of reasons why this movement deterioration might happen.

We tell children, for example, to sit still and not to fidget. We load them up with bags and books, and much of our present educational system seems to conspire to limit their movement opportunities.

For adults, it's often the work environment that conspires to do the same. As grown-ups, we get busy with work, kids, computers, screens, and life. Gradually, these very important movement skills fade into the background. You have probably heard the expression: use it or lose it. Well, it's true.

A lot of people, recognising that they need to do something about this movement deficit, turn to exercise for help. Which is great. Here in the UK, the government issues constantly updated evidence-based guidelines on what they believe people should be doing, eating, and drinking to stay fit and well. I am a great believer in adhering to those guidelines whenever possible.

The difficulty, however, is that all too often exercise alone does not necessarily improve the way that a person is moving through space. In some cases, an enthusiastically embraced exercise regime can cause more harm than good because the person is now adding more weight or miles to a dysfunctional use of their spine.

Certainly, that has often been the case for many of the people who come to me for help.

As a teacher of the Feldenkrais Method®, I don't just work with the 'walking well'. Many of my clients face additional difficulties. It might be that they present with a left-sided stroke, Parkinson's, or are still struggling with their walking after hip or knee replacement surgery. On top of this they may also have a stiff neck, hearing or vision problems, a bad back, or arthritic joints.

In all cases, however, my clients' previous exercise regime, if they had one, failed to address one of the fundamental problems that was affecting their ability to move well: the fact that they were not initiating and expressing balance through their core.

It was to help clients with such disparate needs that I developed the stick technique described below, which is the foundation of the 'Back for the Future' programme.

The stick technique

For the technique to work I needed it to be able to do two things.

Firstly, I needed a technique that would bring lots of healthy and varied movement into my student's spines as efficiently and safely as possible. That was the exercise/movement component.

Secondly, for it to be effective and create real change, I needed a technique that would teach the student how to change the way that they thought about their movement in easily understood terms. The technique would have to give them a series of light-bulb moments that would change the way that the students themselves wanted to move. The feeling and realisation on the part of the client, for example, that if only they used their pelvis and spine to support and to initiate a particular movement, then suddenly their day-to-day life could get a lot easier. This was the skills/learning component.

The use of the stick, as you will discover for yourself, enabled me to achieve these two goals simply, quickly, and efficiently.

The added bonus was that my students, as it turned out, loved working with the sticks. The use of the stick gave them, especially those with real movement challenges such as a stroke, a greater sense of security and made them much more adventurous about exploring more expansive ranges of movement. It made them braver. They were also having a lot of fun interacting with it.

In simple terms, here is how it works: I discovered when working with my clients, particularly my stroke-affected clients, that if I asked them to place the stick in a particular position and asked them to push or pull the stick, I could do all sorts of lovely things to their spines.

If the stick was to their side, for example, and I asked them to reach it out to the side, I could get their spines to side-bend.

Another example would be reaching. By placing the stick on a diagonal and asking the student to reach the stick to the far corner of the room, eventually they would reach the stick so far that their pelvis would begin to respond. Another diagonal would call for a different response from the ribs and spine.

Once the student had practised reaching the stick in this way and realised that reaching the stick had something to do with their spine or pelvis, I could then ask them to repeat the movement but this time begin the movement with the pelvis rather than with the stick.

In the first type of movement, the focus is on the hand on the stick initiating the movement and effectively pulling the spine into a side-bending position (see **Figure A**).

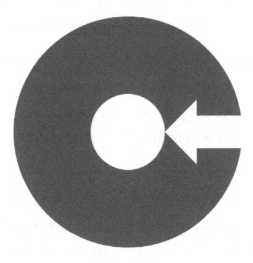

Figure A: A distal-to-core movement. As the hand pushes the stick, for example, the movement travels from the stick and pulls the spine along.

In the second type of movement, the side-bending and reaching of the stick is initiated from their centre (see **Figure B**).

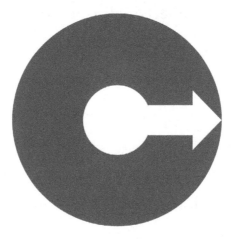

Figure B: A core-to-distal movement. Here the movement is initiated from the centre and travels from the spine to the arm and the stick.

To an outside observer the movement may look the same, but the internal sense of the organisation required is a huge shift for the student. The idea that movement can begin from their core. A light-bulb moment.

To put this more technically, instead of it being a **distal-to-core** (arms to spine) movement it was a **core-to-distal** (spine to arms) movement.

Once this core-to-distal shift had taken place, it could then be used to build up more functionally challenging movements that require shifting through space, such as getting up and out of a chair, walking, or negotiating stairs, which require you to be able to use your core to organise efficient weight transfer.

So, in a nutshell, the stick technique is a method of teaching my students how to reverse the distal-to-core habit. It teaches them how they can begin to activate and use their core to facilitate their movement, not just as part of an exercise but in the carry-over into their daily lives, which in most cases is where it is really needed.

The benefits

Once you learn how to reverse this distal-to-core habit and your movement improves, it has a cascading effect on all aspects of your life, including your:

- Posture
- Core control
- Balance
- Walking
- Breathing
- Self-care
- Self-confidence, and
- Mental wellbeing

All because your movement is synchronised with gravity as opposed to trying to fight it all the time.

In the chapters that follow, you will learn how to use a stick to re-activate the fundamental spinal movements that are the building blocks of your ability to express balance from moment to moment as you move. I think of these building blocks as the ABCs of all good functional movement patterns.

Here's what lies ahead

In **Chapter 1** you will learn the fundamentals of weight-transferring through side-bending. This is done on a chair. Once you have been introduced to the basic pattern of how to do this while keeping your head floating on top of your spine, more complexity will be introduced that will enable you to practise the cross-rotational spinal patterns that are needed for walking.

Chapter 2 takes the spine into different reaching patterns that support the movement of the arms and lay the foundations for more complex weight-transference such as coming to stand or going down a flight of stairs.

Chapter 3 focuses on your abdominal and back muscles. You will learn how to flex and extend the spine in an integrated way that supports the use of the head and eyes and your functional vision. This ability to flex and extend the spine is a key component of being able to organise your posture and balance in standing and making the journey from sitting to standing as effortless as possible.

In **Chapter 4** we take a slight detour and deep-dive into the use of the hips in an exercise that will challenge and improve the mobility of these important joints. You will learn how to connect the legs to the movement of the spine in a way that will support your standing, walking, and ability to go up and down stairs.

Chapter 5 is all about the joy of circles and how you can use the stick to create wonderfully varied movement for the spine. Large circles, small circles, off-centre circles, fast circles, slow circles, one-handed or two-handed circles, the possibilities are endless. Circles will help to integrate the use of the two sides after the asymmetrical explorations in the previous four chapters. The constant weight shifting around the sit bones involved in these circles and the flexibility they bring to the ribs and spine will set you up perfectly for the demands of the following chapters in which we explore the skills required to move through space more dynamically.

Chapter 6 covers the technique of how to get out of a chair and back down effortlessly, using your awareness to harness the power of your legs rather than your arm muscles.

Chapter 7 is the first of two focus chapters and looks at how to improve your walking by integrating the pelvis to find balance and strength as you transition from one leg to another.

In **Chapter 8**, the second focus chapter, you will learn how to negotiate a flight of steps confidently, something of relevance to us all as we get older but especially for anyone who has had hip or knee replacement surgery and who has not yet fully learned how to integrate their new joint into their movement.

Finally, in the **Conclusion** we will look at how you can continue your practice and expand your newly gained movement skills into what matters: your daily life.

In the **list of resources** you will find references to online materials, books, and various organisations that my students and I have found most helpful on our shared movement journey.

What do I need to know before I begin?

In the remainder of this introduction, I will explain how to approach the exercises as a complete beginner and provide a framework of how to build up a lesson that flows from one exercise to another and also tell you what kind of stick and chair works best.

Who is this book for?

Although this book is primarily intended as a reference for the home user, I expect that any movement teacher or exercise professional will find the programme template to be an invaluable guide that they will be able to adapt to structure a class or a lesson for individual clients.

The great advantage for me as a teacher in writing a book about this technique is that it offers me the space to set out the thinking behind the exercises. As a teacher, I have always found that if a student understands why I am asking them to move the stick in a particular way and how it can help them to improve their functional movement then they are much more likely to be engaged with it. You will therefore find quite a lot of explanation within each chapter.

How to approach the programme?

The sequence of the chapters mirrors the way I teach these movements in class. We start with the all-important side-bending and then move on to other functional movement patterns. Each chapter therefore builds upon the previous chapters. My advice to you would be to follow through the material in the order that it is presented.

Chapters 1 to 6 cover the fundamentals, and in a typical class I will teach exercises from each of these chapters in the sequence given. Chapters 7 and 8 deal with specific functions: walking and going up and down stairs. I will only teach this material in class once my students have had plenty of time to practise the ABCs of movement in the earlier chapters.

My advice therefore would be to focus initially on the material in Chapters 1 to 6 and in the sequence that it is presented.

Chapters 1 and 2 are asymmetrical in the sense that we are working the right and left sides with just one hand on the stick. One way of exploring the material in these chapters would be to do each exercise and then switch to the other side. If you would like to do that as you explore the material, then that would be a valid approach, but my preferred method in class is to cover all the material in Chapters 1 and 2 to one side and then repeat the relevant exercises with the stick in the other hand. This helps to create a flowing class and sets up a very nice contrast that helps the students to process the changes that they may be feeling.

A typical class structure therefore would be:

Chapters 1 and 2 with stick in right hand (Figure C).

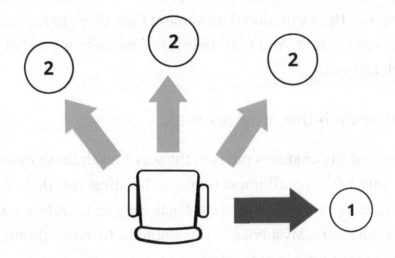

Figure C: The sequence with the stick in the right hand.

1 = Side-bending (Chapter 1), 2 = Long arm reaching (Chapter 2).

And then repeating the exercises in Chapters 1 and 2, but this time with the stick in the left hand (Figure D).

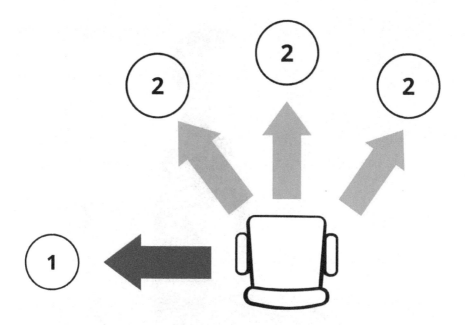

Figure D: The sequence with the stick in the left hand.

1 = Side-bending (Chapter 1), 2 = Long arm reaching (Chapter 2).

Once you have completed the exercises in Chapters 1 and 2 with the stick in the right hand and then repeated them with the stick in the left hand, Chapters 3 to 6 follow in sequence and, depending on time and focus, Chapters 7 and/or 8.

Once you have understood the exercises, it is a simple task to create flowing routines of variable length following the order of the material presented in the chapters adapted to the time you have available.

What kind of chair do I need?

The best kind of chair to use is one that doesn't have arms and has a firm seat.

When you are sitting in the chair with your feet on the floor, the seat should be high enough that your hips are a little bit higher than your knees (Image 1).

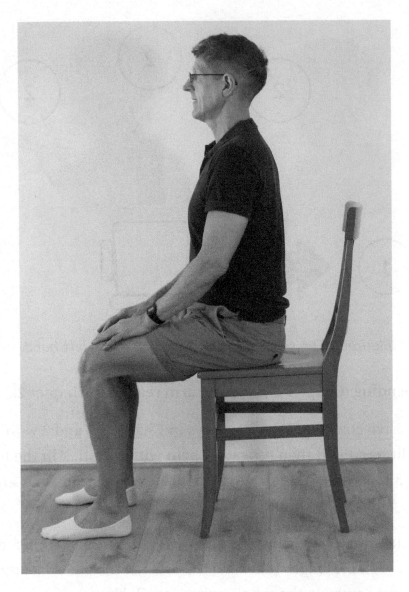

Image 1: Sitting in a chair of the right height. Ideally your hips should be slightly higher than your knees.

If the seat is too low relative to your knees and thighs, it will cause your lower back to round, making it harder for you to sit up on your sit bones without strain. This will inhibit your ability to move well (Image 2).

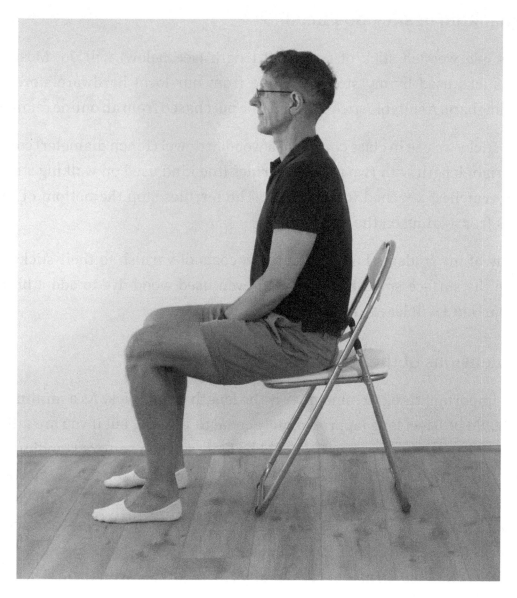

Image 2: Sitting in a chair that is too low. You can see how my hips are lower than my knees and this is causing my back to round.

If you are very tall and struggling to find a high enough chair, some of my taller clients have bought some inexpensive chair height extenders to raise the height of the seat, and you may want to do the same rather than investing in a completely new chair. That's a good idea because you don't want the chair to impede your ability to move.

What kind of stick do I need?

A simple wooden stick of sufficient length (see below) will do. Most of the sticks used by my students come from our local hardware store in Uppingham. A suitable stick can easily be purchased from an online retailer.

The sticks we use in class consist of a wooden dowel (1 inch diameter) cut to the right length with two rubber ferrules (the kind used on walking sticks and crutches) attached to both ends. The ferrules stop the bottom of the stick from sliding on the floor.

Many of my students have added a few coats of varnish to their sticks to keep the surface smooth. Some have even used wood-dye to add a bit of colour, but I will leave any customisation to you.

Dimensions of the stick

The important thing to remember is the length of the stick. As a minimum it should be 5 feet long (approximately equal to 154 cm), but if you are taller than 6 feet (183 cm) your stick should be longer: when you are standing up and the bottom of the stick is placed on the floor, then the top of the stick should be at least as high as the top of your breastbone. For many of my students a precut broomstick works fine. The sticks we use in class don't cost a lot of money. The last stick that I bought, together with the ferrules, cost less that £15. This is another reason why I love working with them. There is no need to pay for lots of expensive equipment.

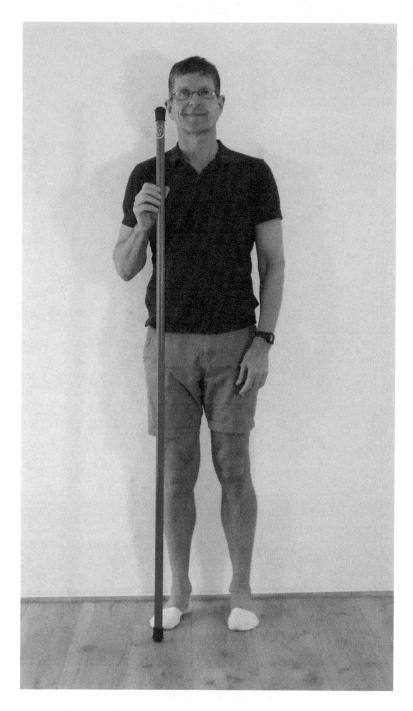

Image 3: The stick should reach at the very least to the top of the breastbone (sternum) in standing—front view. The one I am using in the photographs is cut from a piece of dowel.

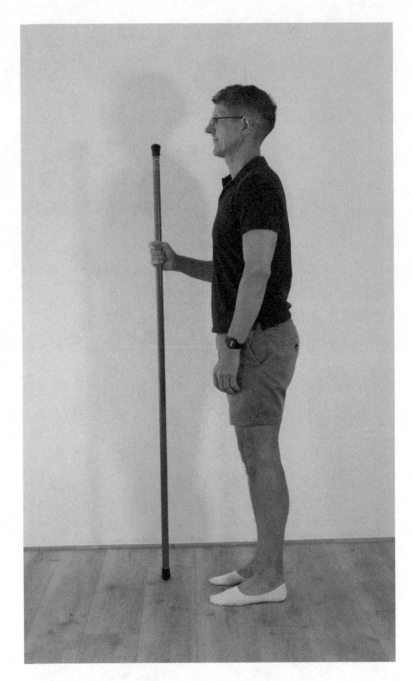

Image 4: Side view.

So, now that you have your stick and chair sorted, let's get started on the journey towards better movement.

1 / SIDE-BENDING—THE KEY TO BALANCE

Your ability to balance well is intimately connected to your ability to side-bend efficiently.

When you can't use your spine and pelvis to side-bend, all sorts of horrible things can happen to your movement, your joints, and your confidence. You become more prone to falls. Perhaps you know someone already who has developed a penguin-like walk, tilting from side to side, as they seek to avoid putting weight on a painful knee or foot. Improving this important functional skill is an absolute must for us all and, as you will discover, easy to do using the stick to help.

Let me give you an example of what I mean by side-bending. It will help you to understand how important it is for our movement.

When I meet a student for the first time, I usually ask them a question. How they answer this question tells us both a lot about how well they are currently moving or not moving.

'Can you show me,' I ask, 'how you would bring your weight on to one buttock or sit bone?'

Perhaps you would like to try this at home before proceeding further to discover what your answer would be?

The student's response usually looks something like this (Image 5).

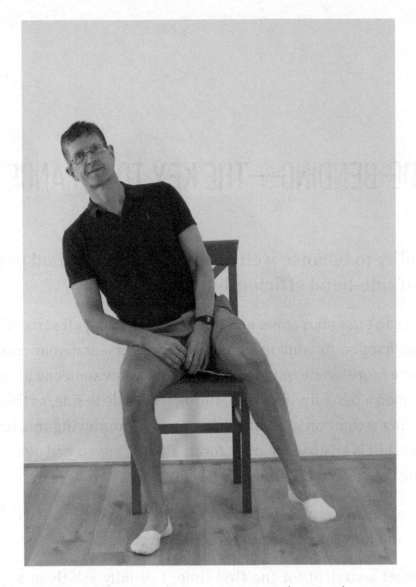

Image 5: This is the typical response I see when I ask someone to show me how they would bring their weight onto one side. Notice how my head has swung in an arc to the right and is now positioned outside the base of support (the chair) and my left foot is lifted.

As opposed to something like this (Image 6).

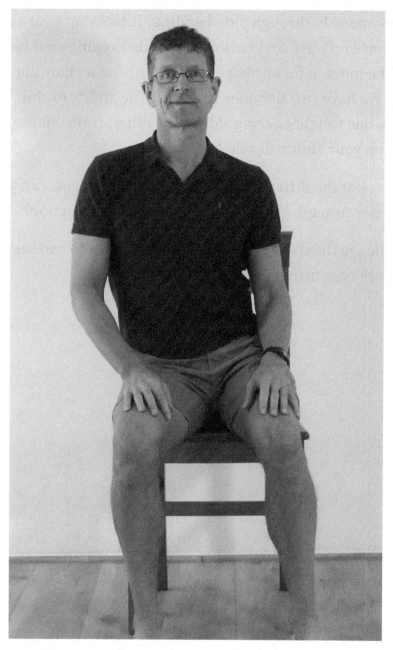

Image 6: Bringing the weight on to the right buttock through side-bending. Here my head is kept over the base of the support and both feet stay on the ground. I am using the whole of my spine and pelvis to transfer weight much more safely.

This ability to bring your weight onto one side through side-bending is a fundamental building block of all good movement. When you bring the weight onto one side through side-bending, it frees up your other side to be able to move forward and backwards while keeping your head upright. This could be moving forwards and backwards on a chair but is also true of walking. We have two sit bones, two legs. The ability to shift weight efficiently from one weight-bearing side to the other, from one leg to another, depends upon your ability to side-bend.

When you look at the difference between the two images, can you see why weight transfer through side-bending is the preferred option?

In the first image the spine is used as if it is a stick. You can see this also in Image 8 where I am using my assistant Boris to help!

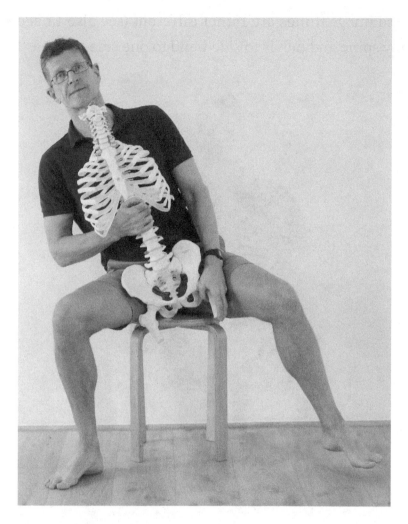

Image 7: The spine being used as a stick to transfer weight.
Notice how my left shoulder is higher than the right.

The person who uses this strategy to transfer their weight is **tilting** their spine. The spine is hardly bending at all. A consequence of this is that the head moves in a large arc from side to side and because the head is being displaced outside the base of the support (here the chair) the person is having to use a lot of muscular effort to stop themselves from falling off the chair. When I see a person doing this in the studio, they are usually also showing signs of tension in their jaw or tongue, and breath. The foot on the opposite side is often lifted to act as a counterweight to prevent the fall.

In the second image things are rather different (see also Image 8 below). I am using my spine and pelvis to side-bend to one side.

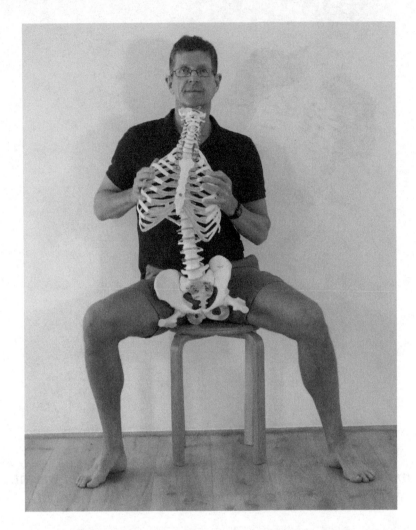

Image 8: With side-bending the whole of the spine is being used to transfer weight. The spine curves over to the right. Notice how my left shoulder is lower than the right.

The huge advantage here is that the head is kept in the middle. It is therefore kept over the base of support. This means that the balance of a person who side-bends is much more dynamically stable than the person who uses a tilt as a strategy to shift their weight. With side-bending the head is supported and therefore the person is able to scan the horizon with their head, eyes, and ears whereas in the previous image the head is 'busy' being used to balance, and its freedom to do other things is compromised.

This may not seem like a big deal when you are sitting in a chair, but you can readily appreciate how important it is in walking.

You will often see people who walk through tilting: the penguin-like waddle mentioned previously. This is quite a common pattern for a person who has a knee or hip problem. They compensate to avoid bearing weight down into an arthritic and painful joint. The head and shoulders tilt from side to side as they try to make progress forward. Their balance is under constant threat, and they quickly become exhausted by the extra effort involved in moving. Weight is not passing through their joints but being cast from side to side, and it's perhaps not surprising that the rest of their system is put under strain and that they begin to suffer from a host of other ailments such as a bad back, stiff neck and shoulders.

One of the things that inspired me to develop the stick programme was my experience of working with so many people who have had successful hip or knee replacement surgery but who have continued to walk with this grinding tilt because they haven't been taught how to integrate their new joint into more efficient movement patterns. They were still walking as if they hadn't had their surgery at all, still unable to fully enjoy their lives.

However, it is not just a person's walking and balance that will improve if you can change the way that they weight-transfer through side-bending. As a skill, side-bending is also a component of your ability to reach for an object without straining your neck and shoulders, to roll out of bed, to get dressed, to wash, to wipe your bottom or even to get easily in or out of your car.

So, now that you have understood its importance, let's begin to explore how you can use the stick on a chair to learn how to effectively weight-transfer through side-bending.

Exercise 1: Weight transference through tilting

To make the distinction between tilting and side-bending crystal clear, we are in fact going to begin with tilting.

Come to sit at the front edge of your chair with your feet on the floor and with your feet and knees at least hip distance apart (Image 9).

Place the stick to your right and take hold of it with your right hand as comfortably high as you can without putting strain on your shoulder. Relax the jaw. Breathe comfortably.

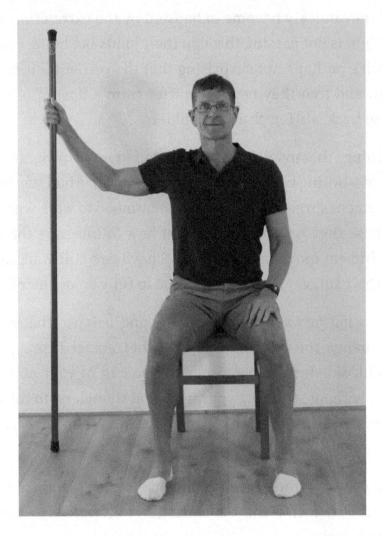

Image 9: Exercise 1 start position with stick on right. Viewed from front.

Looking from the side, the stick shouldn't be too far forward but equally not too far back (Image 10).

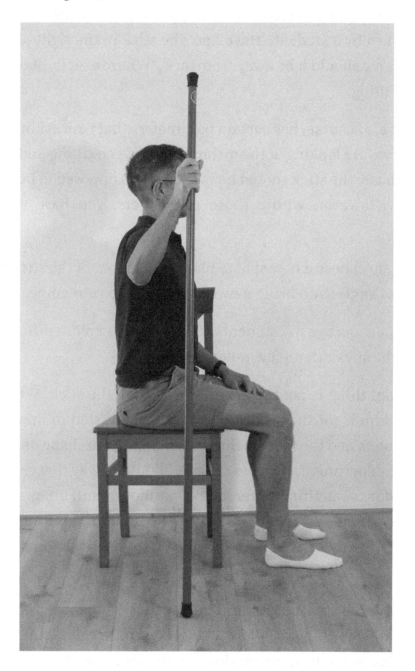

Image 10: Exercise 1 start position viewed from the side.

"Have I got the stick in the right place?"

Now here's an important sidenote that applies to all the exercises. I sometimes get asked by a student, 'Have I got the stick in the right place?', 'How many inches etc should it be away from me?', 'Where exactly should it be?'—that kind of thing.

Each exercise, of course, has certain parameters that I am asking you to observe. Here we are looking at the difference between tilting and side-bending, so obviously the stick should be to the side as opposed to being behind or in front. However, within those parameters, you have a wealth of possibilities.

Every time you choose a new spot to place the bottom of the stick it is going to create new angles and bring new movement into your spine.

That's why I encourage my students to constantly explore different places to position the stick after a few repetitions.

The important thing is not the precise location of the stick. What is much more important is for the student to become interested in how the placement of the stick and the movements are changing the shape of their spine. So please do experiment. Become curious about the way that each position of the stick does something different to your movement. Enjoy the sense of the variety of movement. We are looking to bring change into your spine, to make it more flexible and supple and not get hung up on doing things 'the right way'.

Begin to reach the stick out to the side. Do this a few times, slowly, and if you are not already doing so, allow your head to follow the spine (Image 11). This is, in fact, what most people do to begin with anyway. They tilt. See if you can notice what is happening to your spine.

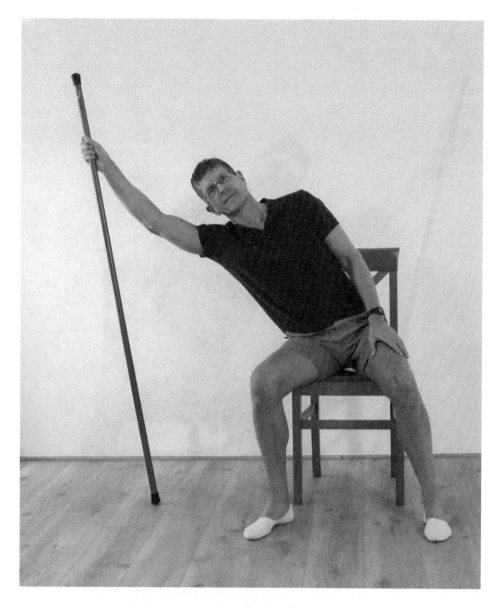

Image 11: Tilting to the right, head following the stick.

You should reach far enough to the side that you can clearly feel that your left buttock has become light.

If necessary, you can always pause to the side and check that you truly have brought your weight on to the right by sliding your left palm under your left buttock. If you can do that easily, *'bingo!'* You have successfully transferred your weight onto the right buttock through tilting.

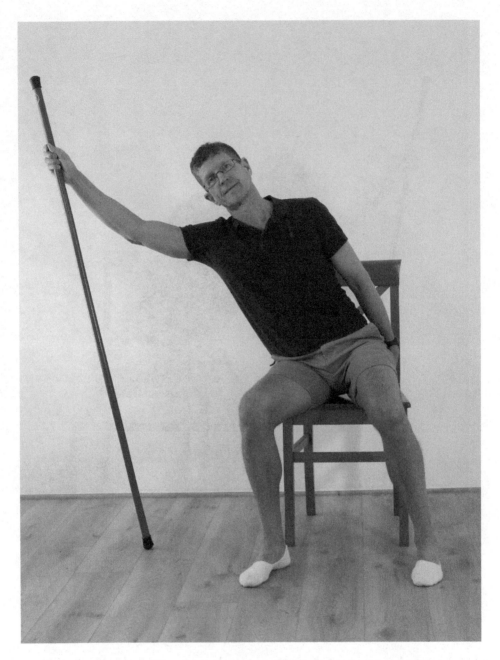

Image 12: Tilting to the right, checking with the left palm that the left buttock has become light.

Repeat this tilting to the side several times, allowing the head to follow the stick until it becomes very clear to you that you have shifted the weight onto the right sit bone. Try a few different places for the stick. Then move on to the next exercise.

"Should I try this to the other side now?"

When I teach these exercises in class, the sequence I usually follow, as mentioned in the introduction, is to perform all the exercises in Chapters 1 and 2 with the stick in the same hand. Here we are working with the stick in the right hand. I then repeat the same sequence of exercises with the stick in the left hand to the other side.

This creates a nice flowing sequence, saves time, and helps to create a contrast in the two sides. I would encourage you to do the same, but this is a personal choice for you to make and will depend on the time you have and how you wish to approach your own explorations and learning.

Switching from one side to the other after each of the exercises in Chapters 1 and 2 is a perfectly valid strategy but, in a class setting, tends to be too 'fussy' and takes up valuable time.

Exercise 2: Tilting into side-bending

We can now use this ability to tilt to learn how to side-bend.

Tilt to the right once more, following the stick with the head, and see if you can stay there, tilted to the right.

Allow the stick to linger to the right, and begin to come back by lifting the head up and over to the left to return your weight onto your two sit bones, as if you were heading a football (Image 13).

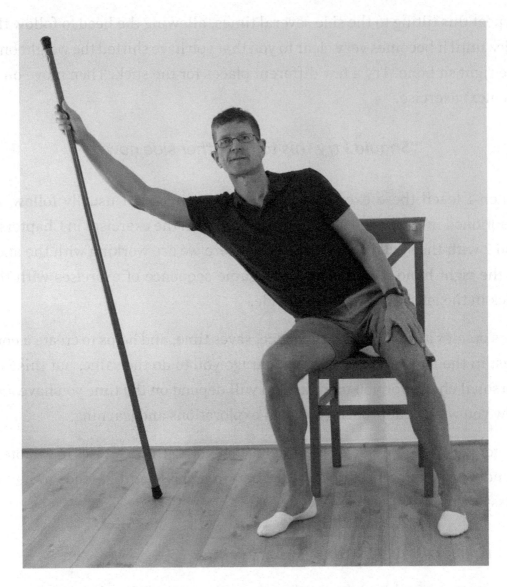

Image 13: Exercise 2. From the tilted position, allow the stick to linger to the right and begin to lift the head up and over to the left.

If you go slowly and pay attention to how the shape of your spine is changing as you begin to lift up through the head, you will notice how the ribs underneath the left armpit concertina together as the spine follows the head to bring you back onto the two sit bones (Image 14).

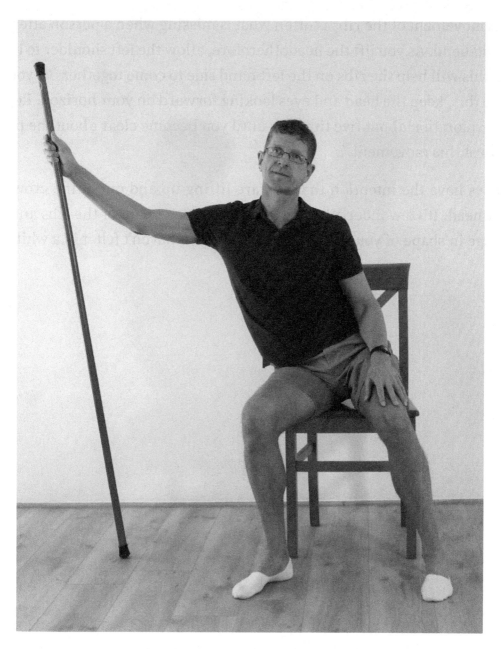

Image 14: Exercise 2. Notice that as my head is moving over to the left away from the stick, the left shoulder is now lower that the right. You can't see through my shirt, but this means that the ribs on my left-hand side are closing together to facilitate the coming back. My left-hand side is shorter than my right, but you can see from the space under my left buttock that my weight is still on my right sit bone. My spine has changed shape from a straight line to a curve.

This movement of the ribs is often what is missing when a person attempts to side-bend. As you lift the head, therefore, allow the left shoulder to lower and this will help the ribs on the left-hand side to come together. As you explore this, keep the head and eyes looking forward on your horizon. Repeat the exploration about five times or until you become clear about the possibility of this movement.

Always have the intention that you are lifting up and out of the crown of your head. It's a wonderful thing to feel this movement of the ribs and the change in shape of your spine, especially if you haven't felt it in a while.

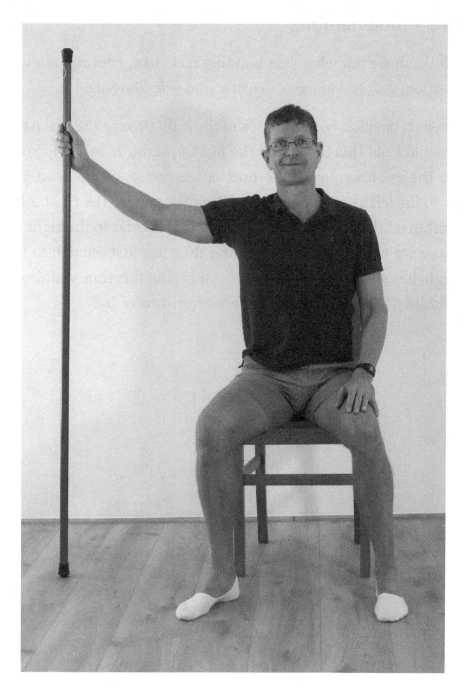

Image 15: Arriving back on to both sit bones.

Exercise 3: **Side-bending**

Now that you have felt what side-bending feels like, coming into it from a tilted position, it's time to move directly into side-bending.

From the start position with the stick to the right (Image 15), reach the stick out to the right but this time keep the head upright. It will help you if you can have the intention, as in the previous exercise, of the head going up and over to the left as your weight and the stick shift to the right. Allow the ribs to soften on the left. The stick will not move as far to the right as it did when you were tilting. You are reaching the stick just enough to feel that your weight has shifted onto the right buttock, but this time your head stays in the middle. This is the pattern we are after (Image 16):

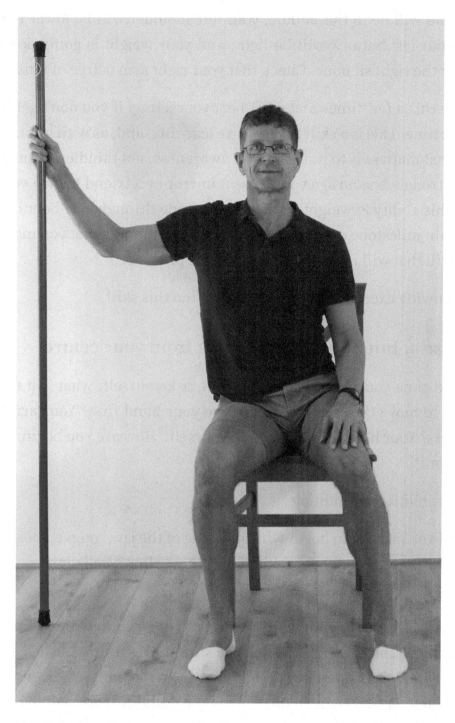

Image 16: Side-bending to my right, keeping my head in the middle. Notice how the left shoulder is lower than the right. The left shoulder and the left side of the pelvis have come together and my weight is on the right buttock.

Your head will be in the middle, your left shoulder will be lower than the right, your left buttock will be light, and your weight is going down and through the right sit bone. Check that your right arm is free of tension.

Practise this a few times and don't beat yourself up if you don't get it right the first time. This is a skill that you are learning, and, as with learning any skill, what matters is to practise with awareness, not mindless repetition. I would strongly encourage you to use a mirror or a friend to give you feedback. This ability to weight-transfer to one side through side-bending is an important milestone on your way to improving the way that you move, and it is a skill that will improve over time with practice.

The following exercise will help you to refine this skill.

Exercise 4: Initiating side-bending from your centre

The next time you side-bend to the right, ask yourself: what is it that you do **first** to move the stick? Do you move your hand first? Your arm? Your shoulders? Your head? Your ribs? Ask yourself: 'How are **you** beginning the movement?'

The possibilities are multiple.

For some people, it can begin with a tensing of the jaw, tongue, toes, a holding of the breath or any combination of those. Don't be judgmental about this, but do be curious.

Commonly, a person will begin the movement with the hand that is holding the stick. The grip tightens and the stick moves as it is pushed away by the hand, and the movement then travels from the hand, through the arm to the shoulder and then so on. This is the **distal-to-core pattern** that we spoke about in the introduction in which movement is initiated from the periphery (here your right hand) to the centre (your spine).

To really begin to turbo-charge your movement, however, we want to re-fine your ability to initiate the movement from your core and specifically the pelvis.

Here's why: all your big powerful muscles are attached to your pelvis. They include your abdominals, back muscles, gluteal muscles, and leg muscles.

The further you move away from the spine towards your hands and feet, the smaller the muscles get.

You can think of this as the pelvis being responsible for doing the heavy lifting while the smaller muscles help with fine motor control and detail.

If the pelvis isn't playing its usual part in your movement, then it can dis-tort everything you do movement-wise and in some cases act as a serious deadweight.

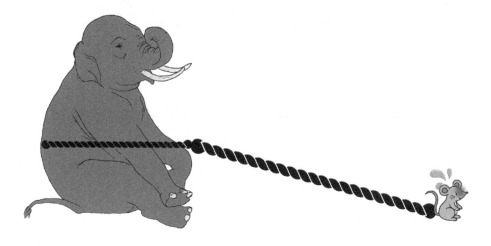

Figure E: The distal-to-core pattern. The mouse of course represents your smaller, peripheral muscles trying to move the core.

The smaller muscles, which are really meant for activities that require finer control, are often then called upon to do more of the heavy lifting (Figure E).

If, therefore, we can bring the power of the pelvis 'online' and initiate movement from this area, you will be better at coordinating your movement and balance and using your stronger muscles to support the use of the limbs (Figure F).

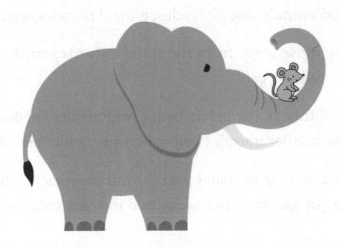

Figure F: When movement is initiated from the core, your bigger, more powerful muscles support the use of the limbs.

Let's try it.

One way of thinking of initiating the movement of side-bending from the pelvis is to think of beginning it by hitching up, in this case, the left hip. If you look again at the photograph of me in Image 16 above, you will see that my left side is shorter than the right. The hip is 'hitched' up, and the left shoulder and left hip have come closer together.

In a way, this idea of 'hitching up' the hip will do the trick, and it's a cue that I sometimes give my students to help them grasp the idea of starting a movement from the pelvis. It's a feeling that's very familiar to mums and dads who have had to carry an infant. Try it and see. Initiate the side-bending to the right by hitching up the left hip. It usually works for most people to kick-start the movement from the pelvis.

There is a problem with this cue, however, and we can make it much better by using a cue that more closely incorporates the pattern of weight transference that we need in standing and walking.

The problem with simply thinking of hitching up the hip is that it often causes strain in the other hip.

In standing or walking, something we cover in later chapters, it's not a question of hitching up one hip to bring your weight onto the other leg but of actively pouring your weight down through the weight-bearing leg and hip joint. You can think of it as a reaching down from the pelvis into the weight-bearing hip and leg, and that is what we want to practise on the chair with the stick.

Here is a visualisation that I often use with my students and that may help you with this.

Imagine that there is a grape underneath your right sit bone and think that you are reaching down with your right sit bone or buttock to squash the grape (Figure G). As you reach down with your right sit bone, the left sit bone will lift. But this lift comes from pressing the right sit bone into the seat of the chair. The left side responds to the movement as opposed to initiating it.

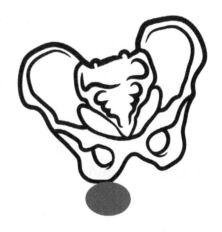

Figure G: Rather than think of lifting up the left side of the pelvis, think that you are reaching down with the right side to squash an imaginary ball or grape.

Once you get the idea that the transference of weight is a reach down rather than a lift, you will be amazed at what a difference this can make to your movement both in the chair and, as we will see in later chapters, in standing.

Take your time to practise this. It requires you to think about how you are initiating your movement and to bring a certain intention to it. Forming and expressing this intention is the key to change.

Once you have become more familiar with the idea and embodiment of side-bending, it's time to add some complexity and variations to your new-found ability because in 3D life we don't just side-bend like fish to move. We need to combine side-bending with rotational forward and backwards movements. This is what we will explore in the exercises ahead.

Exercise 5: Side-bending while turning the head

Some people's neck and shoulders are so stiff that, if they need to look at an object to their side, they have to turn the whole of their torso and head as a block to bring the item into their field of vision. This makes such a person vulnerable to falls and, as you can imagine, exposes them to other risks. For example, he or she cannot react easily while waiting to cross a road to see if there is a vehicle or cyclist approaching at speed from one side. The following exercise explores your ability to differentiate the movement of your head and eyes while also side-bending.

With the stick in your right hand, side-bend as in the previous exercise to bring your weight onto your right buttock initiating the movement as best you can from your pelvis (squashing the grape!).

As you side-bend to the right, look with your head and eyes to the left (Image 17).

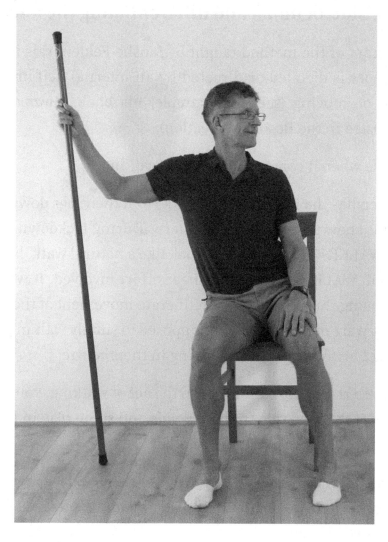

Image 17: Side-bending to the right, looking with head and eyes to the left.

When you return to the centre, bring your head and eyes to look forward again.

Repeat several times until you can do this without holding your breath and reduce any unnecessary tension. Check that your jaw is relaxed and that the stick-holding hand is as soft as possible. Try to make this a single smooth movement rather than thinking of first side-bending and then moving the head.

Then move on to the next exercise.

Exercise 6: Side-bending and differentiating the knee

A central tenant of the method taught by Moshe Feldenkrais is that a person's movement is dictated or directed by an internal 'self-image' of how they should be moving (see, for example, his book, *'Awareness Through Movement'*, listed in the Resources section).

This is so true when it comes to a person's walking.

A person often has the idea that they walk from their legs downwards and, boy, does this show up in their gait pattern. During lockdown, I often saw people out 'WALKING'. It often didn't look like a natural walk, but you knew they were out 'WALKING' from the sheer effort involved. It was as if they were announcing through the very deliberate movement of their arms and legs that they were out 'WALKING' as opposed to simply walking. The limbs were moving but nothing was happening in their centre.

However, if you reflect for a moment on the act of walking, you will quickly come to realise the vital role that the pelvis and spine play in the transference of your weight from one leg to another.

Fluid contra-lateral walking, with the opposite arm and leg moving in time, is a whole-body event that incorporates side-bending, rotation, flexion, and extension of the spine.

In this exercise, and the ones that follow, we will practise your ability to differentiate the movement of the pelvis from the chest and head while side-bending, providing a valuable opportunity to develop the same skill set that you need when off your chair.

With the stick to your right and in your right hand, side-bend to bring your weight onto the right buttock as before (think 'squash the grape') and then stay there with your weight on the right sit bone and your head and eyes looking forward on your horizon.

Make sure you are breathing and that the jaw and stick-holding hand are free of tension. Your left buttock should not be touching the seat of the chair.

Keep your left foot planted where it is on the floor, and begin to move your left knee a little bit forward and a little bit backward in space (Image 18).

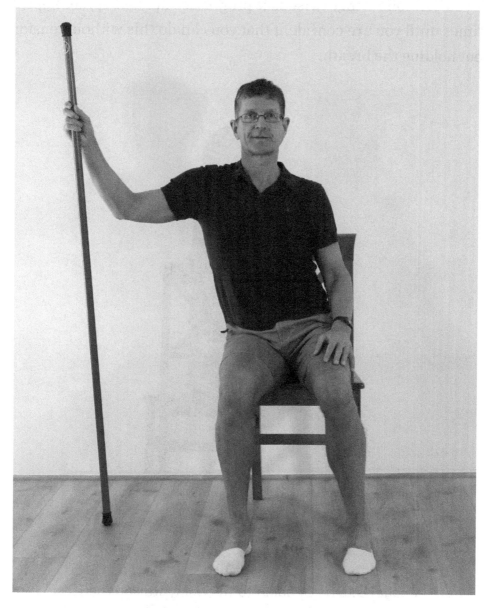

Image 18: Side-bending to the right, staying there, and moving the left knee forward and back. Front view.

The knee goes straight forward and back. Not out to the side or to the mid-line.

Notice that to take the knee forward and back, it's the left side of the pelvis that is moving forward and back and because the pelvis is moving in this way, we are therefore introducing a twist into the spine (Images 19 and 20). See if you can follow that twist as it progresses up your spine. Repeat several times until you are confident that you can do this without tension and without holding the breath.

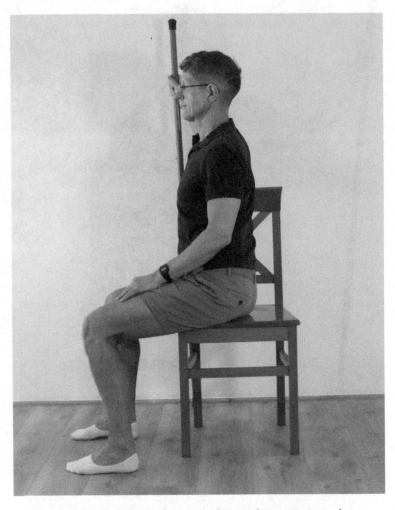

Image 19: Side-bending to the right, staying there, and moving the left knee forward. Side view.

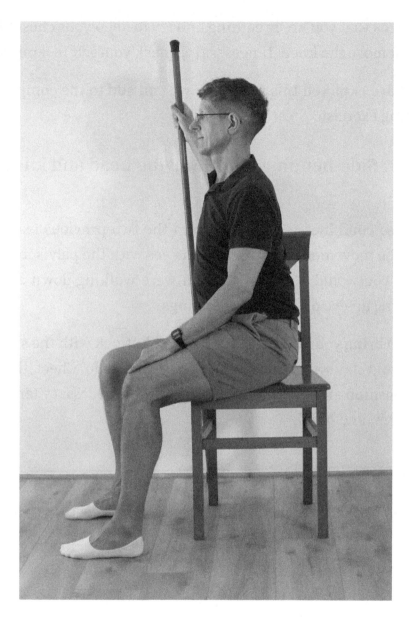

Image 20: Side-bending to the right, staying there, and moving the left knee backwards. Side view.

Now, one thing to watch for when you are doing this exercise is to check what is happening to your chest. If you discover that your chest and shoulders are also turning with the movement of the knee, that would mean that you are not differentiating the movement of the pelvis from the rest of the spine. If that is happening with you, slow things down, make the movement smaller, check that you are breathing and try to keep your chest facing forward as you move the knee. If necessary, check yourself in a mirror.

Once you have explored this variation, we can add to the complexity with the following exercise.

Exercise 7: Side-bending while moving head and knee together

This exercise combines movements from the two previous exercises and integrates the movement of the head and eyes with the pelvis in side-bending, just as you would need to do if you were walking down a busy high street keeping an eye on your surroundings.

Side-bend to bring your weight onto the right buttock with the stick in your right hand and stay with your weight on the right side. Check that you can be in this position and breathe and reduce any unnecessary tension in the jaw, right arm, and hand.

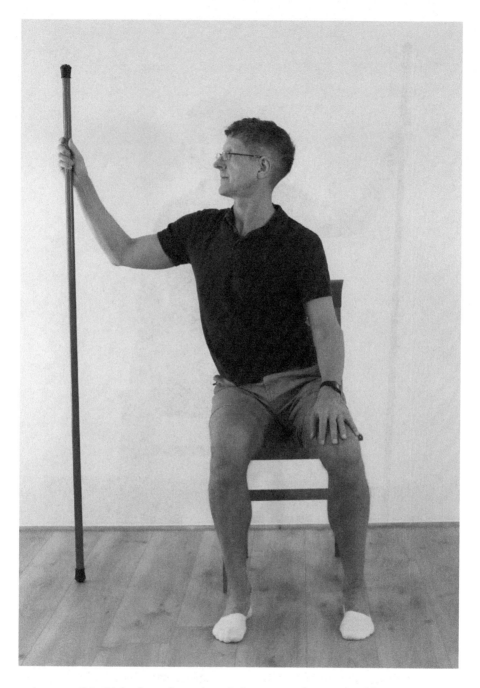

Image 21: Side-bend to the right, stay there, and look to the right as the left knee moves forwards. Front view.

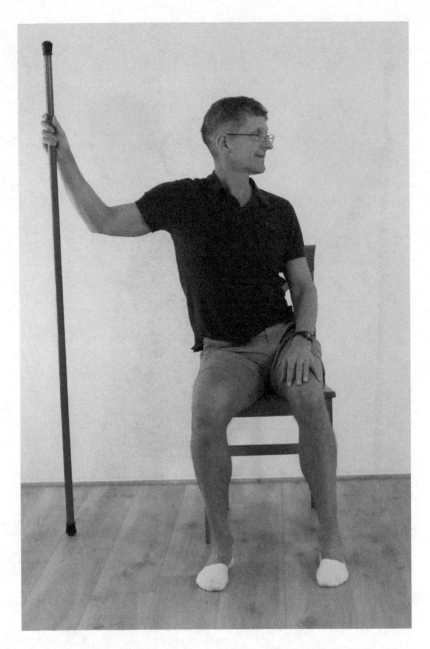

Image 22: Side-bend to the right, stay there, look to the left as the left knee moves backwards. Front view.

As you move your left knee forward and backwards, keep your chest facing the front, and begin to turn your head and eyes left and right in a way that is synchronised with the movement of the knee.

In other words, as your left knee moves forwards, turn the head and eyes to the right, and as your knee moves backwards, turn the head and eyes to your left. Keep your eyes scanning the horizon rather than looking down at the floor (Images 21 to 24).

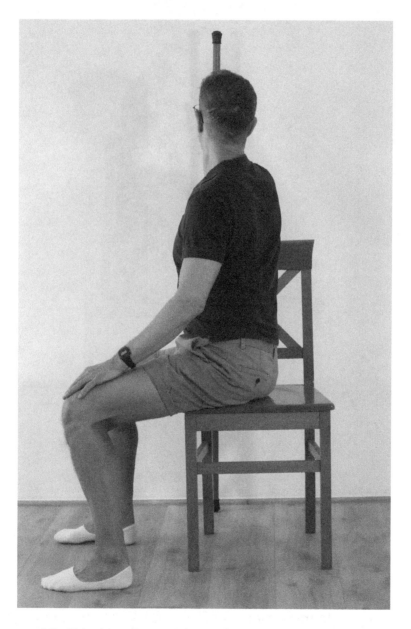

Image 23: Side-bending to the right, staying there, and as the left knee moves forward, looking to the right. Side view.

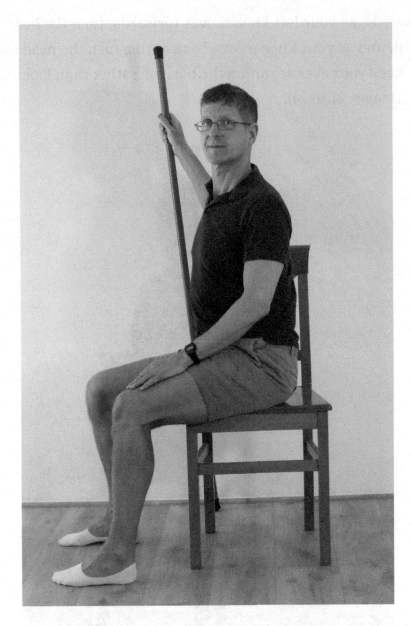

Image 24: Side-bending to the right, staying there, and as the left knee moves backward, looking to left. Side view.

Once again, see if you can think of this as being a single movement as opposed to two separate movements of first your knee and then your head. In other words, notice how you are moving from your centre.

Repeat until you can do this smoothly and with a minimum of tension.

Things get a little bit more complicated in the next variation.

Exercise 8: Side-bending with opposition of the knee and head

Judging from the smiles I see whenever I teach the following exercise to my students, they really enjoy it. It's a lot of fun to try out and is a little bit like the children's game of patting your head while rubbing your tummy.

It's a movement puzzle that introduces greater complexity for your brain to cope with and therefore requires a higher level of coordination. As your nervous system is engaged in solving the puzzle, it means your brain must let go of holding patterns that interfere with your ability to move. The key to solving the puzzle is to pay attention to your breath and to slow things down.

Side-bend to the right with the stick in your right hand and stay there.

This time as you move your left knee forward and back, turn the head and eyes **in opposition** to the movement of the knee.

In other words, as the knee goes forward, look to your left and as your knee goes backwards, look to your right.

Keep your head and eyes at all times looking on the horizon (Images 25 to 28).

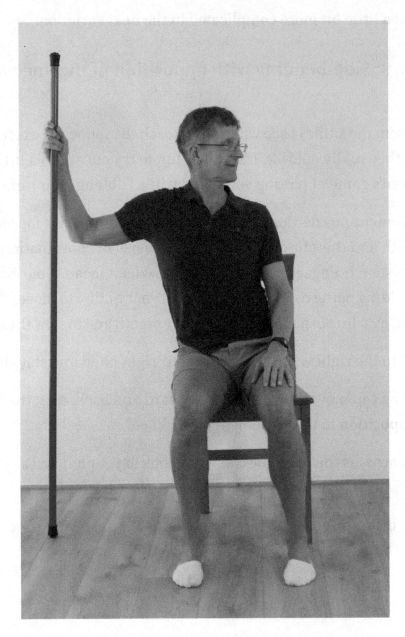

Image 25: As the left knee moves forward, look to the left. Front view.

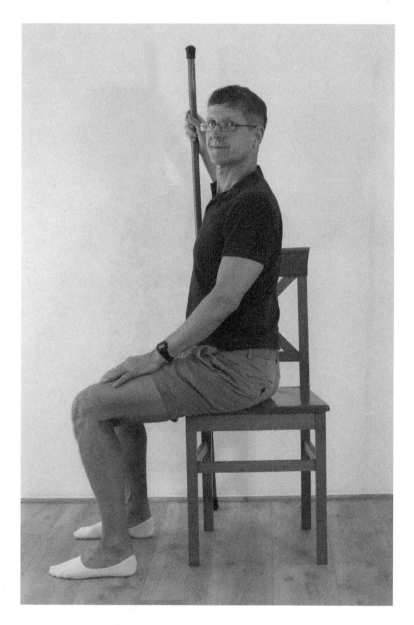

Image 26: Side view of the head and knee moving in opposition. Knee forward, head to the left.

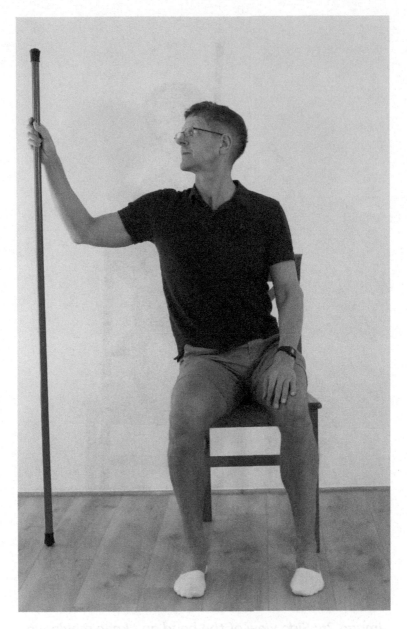

Image 27: As the left knee moves backwards, look to the right. Front view.

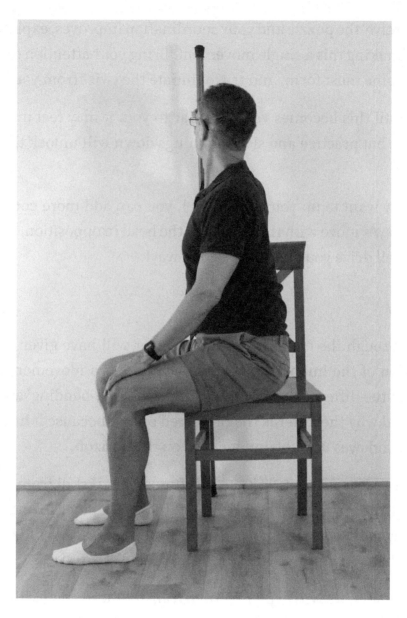

*Image 28: Side view of oppositional movement:
left knee back, head to the right.*

Repeat several times.

Once you 'solve' the puzzle and your coordination improves, explore the possibility of making this a single movement. Bring your attention to the shape that your spine must form, and try to initiate the twist from your centre.

Practise until this becomes very familiar to you. It may feel impossible to begin with, but practice and slowing things down will unlock the skill and your spine.

If you really want to up your skills level, you can add more complexity by having the eyes move with the knees but the head in opposition. Attempting this may well drive you crazy—in a good way!

Summary

Working through the exercises in this chapter will have given you a deep appreciation of the importance of side-bending as a movement skill. You have learnt the difference between 'tilting' and 'side-bending' as a balance strategy and why the latter is the preferred option because it helps to keep your head and eyes upright and focused on the horizon.

You have also learnt how to initiate this fundamental skill from your pelvis ('squashing the grape') and how to maintain your balance to one side while introducing more complex movements for the spine, head, and eyes. These are skills that will improve with time and practice.

In later chapters, we will explore how to transfer these new skills into walking, but for the moment give yourself a huge pat on the back. You are ready to move on to the next vital skill: how to support the movement of your arms from the spine.

2 / REACHING: HOW TO USE THE SPINE TO SUPPORT THE ARMS

If you have ever tried to drive a car forward and forgotten to take the hand-brake off, as I have done on occasion, you will know that it's not easy to drive very far.

In fact, keeping the brakes on while trying to drive away is a bad idea and a very good way of messing up your brakes and engine. It's even harder to move forward if you have also left the gear in reverse. Harder still if you haven't even turned on the ignition.

One solution might be to get out of the car and try to lift the front and pull your vehicle forward. But that would be stupid, wouldn't it? I couldn't do it and even the attempt would mess up my back and neck (Image 29).

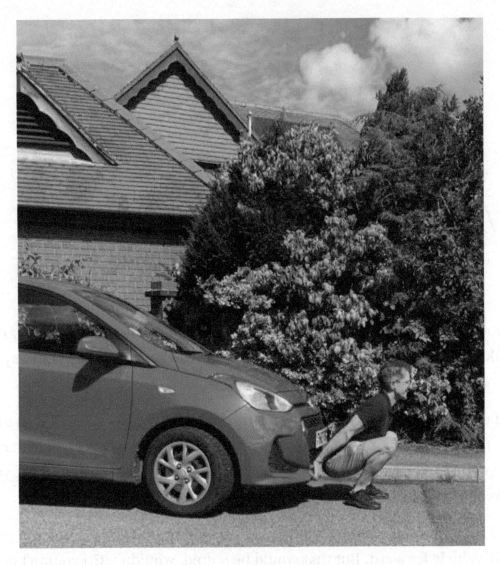

Image 29: As you can see, I am not going to get very far with this!

The obvious solution, you would think, would be to turn on the ignition, put the car in gear, and take off the handbrake. What's true of the car is also true of how you use your arms. Simple really, if you want to make life easier.

Let me explain what I mean, and then show you some exercises that will help you to take the brakes off your arms.

We take our hands and arms for granted so much that we forget sometimes just how amazing they are. When we made the evolutionary journey of coming up onto our hind limbs and moving around on two legs, we began to organise our movement around the vertical axis of our spine. This helped to free up our arms to enable us to do all the amazing things that we do with them.

Functionally, the arms and hands play a vital role in our ability to look after ourselves. Think about how you get dressed, how you wash, how you go to the toilet, how you feed yourself, how you move, how you balance, and how you look after your children or grandchildren, your garden, your pets, your home. For many people their ability to work is dependent on the healthy use of their arms: dentists, mechanics, hairdressers, barbers, musicians etc. Life can be devastating and so much more difficult when the functional use of an arm is lost. So, how we use them matters.

The next time you are in a coffee shop, supermarket, office, or any situation where you can look at what people are doing, without appearing weird, notice how the people around you are reaching for something.

If the person is sitting at a table or desk and going to reach for something, their reaching may well look something like this (Image 30).

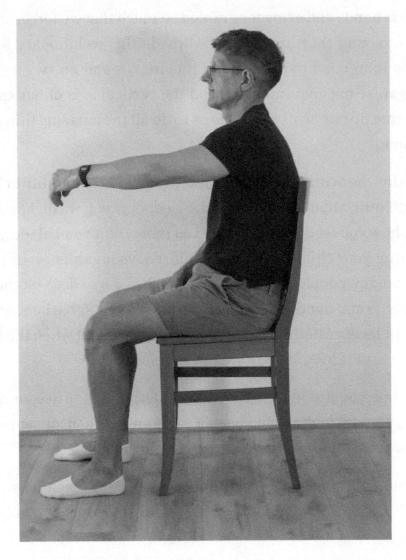

Image 30: A very typical example of reaching for an object. The arm is being lifted forward and the back is doing nothing to help. The equivalent of the engine being switched off and the gear left in reverse.

It could however look something like this (Image 31).

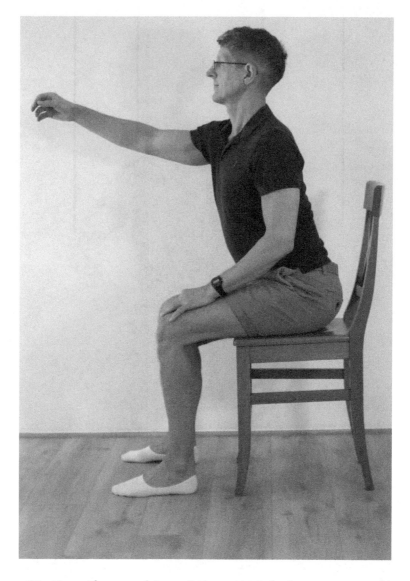

Image 31: Here the reaching of the arm is being supported by and initiated from the core. The engine is switched on and in gear.

In the first image, I am not using my back and pelvis to support the movement of the arm. In the second image, I am.

In the first of the two images, because I am not supporting the reach of my arm with the spine and pelvis, I am effectively trying to lift my arm to bring it forward. Rather like a puppet master would use the strings of a puppet to lift its limbs (Image 32).

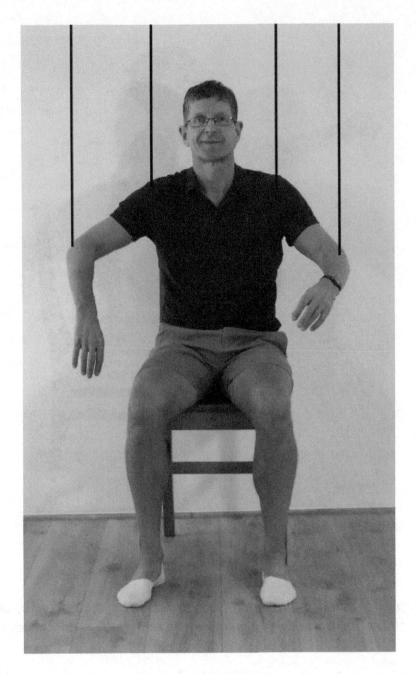

Image 32: Here, because I am not engaging my centre to move my arms, I have to lift my arms to move them, rather like a puppet is moved, only it is the smaller muscles of my neck and shoulders that are having to be substituted for strings.

One of the consequences of this is that, instead of using the back to support the reach, a person with this habit of self-use is using muscles that attach to the head and neck to move the arm. They are lifting the arm against the pull of gravity and the arms are heavy. These smaller, shorter neck and shoulder muscles can then become perpetually contracted, shorter, tighter, and overworked.

Over time, this dysfunctional misuse can lead to neck and shoulder issues as the mobility of this area is reduced. It's perhaps not surprising that there appears to be an epidemic of neck pain complaints. A person suffering in this way will often try exercises or treatment that targets those muscles in an attempt to stretch or strengthen them, but the underlying pattern of misuse remains, and the neck problem keeps on repeating itself.

The 'self-image' such a person with this puppet habit often has is that their arms begin at the top of the long upper arm bones (the humerus) and their arms are something to be lifted as opposed to it being a part of them that can be supported in their movement from the spine and pelvis through effective weight transference.

The exercises that follow will help you to construct a different self-image.

As mentioned in the previous chapter, my approach in teaching these exercises in class is to keep the stick in one hand as you explore all the exercises in sequence before switching to the other side. The instructions therefore focus on using the stick in the right hand. If you are working with the stick in the left hand, simply mirror the instructions to suit.

Exercise 9: Reaching on the diagonal—first angle

Sit at the front edge of your chair with the feet and knees shoulder-width apart and hold the stick in your right hand as comfortably high as you can without putting strain into your shoulder or arm. Always try to keep your grip on the stick as soft as possible, with the arm long but not locked.

Place the bottom end of the stick on the floor in line with the direction that your right knee is facing (Image 33).

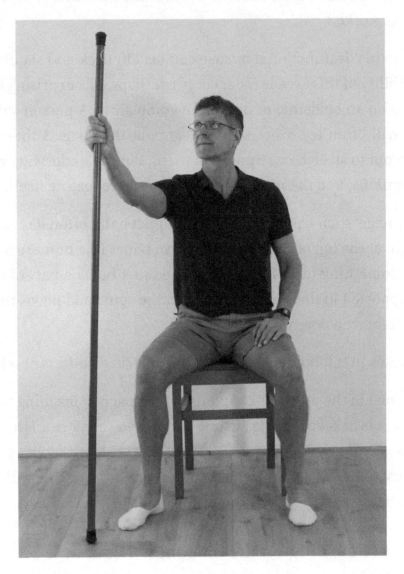

Image 33: Start position for the first angle. Notice that my arm is long but not locked out at the elbow. If you tend to hyperextend at the elbow and therefore impact the shoulder, you will need to remember to keep the elbow soft.

If you were sitting at the centre of a clock with 12 o'clock directly in front of you, 3 o'clock to your right, and 9 o'clock to your left, then the stick would be somewhere between 1 and 2 o'clock (**Figure H**).

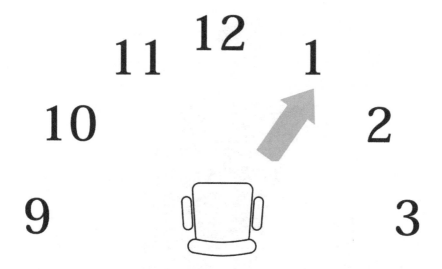

Figure H: First angle. The angle shown here is somewhere between 1 and 2 o'clock, but I would encourage you to try several different angles in this area of our clock. Each angle will ask your spine, ribs, and all the associated muscles and tissue to respond in a different way. Another variable that you could explore is to have the bottom of the stick a little bit further away from you.

Reach the stick away from you on the angle. It's as if you are reaching to touch the far corner of your room.

As you reach the stick, look up at the top of the stick or, at the very least, above the position of your hand on the stick. Keep the tip of your nose lined up with the stick (Image 34).

When you have reached as far forward as you comfortably can, return to the start position, bringing your head and eyes to look on the horizon.

Do this several times to get used to the movement.

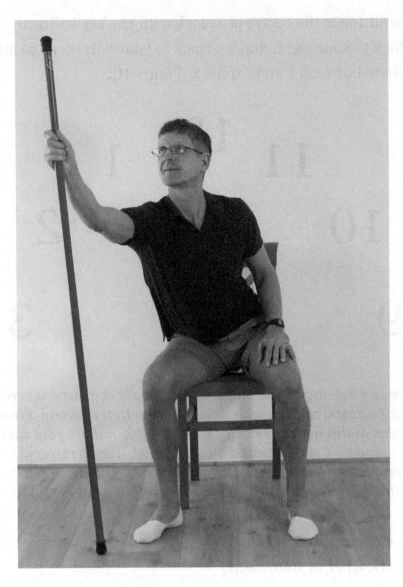

Image 34: Reaching to the right-hand corner of the room (first angle). Remember to use your vision to help you with the movement. Look up at the top of the stick as you reach the stick forward and then return the head and eyes to the horizon as you return. If you look at the image closely you will see that there is 'daylight' under my left buttock area as the left side of the pelvis lifts. Notice how my weight has shifted onto the right buttock and my left side is 'shorter' than my right.

As you explore this movement notice what happens to your spine.

As you reach forward and far enough, the spine is 'pulled' along with the movement. The front of the body lengthens which is why it is important to look up. There is side-bending of the spine and your weight shifts onto the right sit bone. Can you feel how the ribs on the left-hand side come together as your weight shifts onto the right-hand side and how the left-hand side of the pelvis lifts? The left sit bone becomes light as you reach away on the diagonal (Image 35).

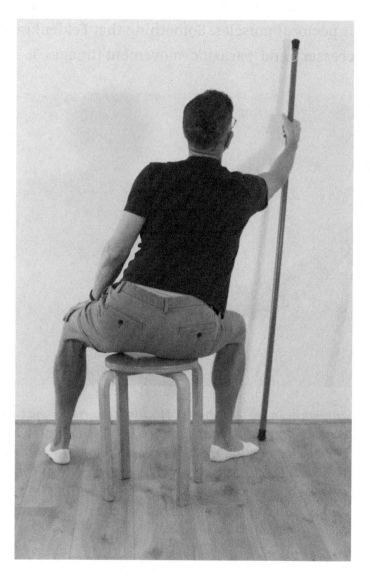

Image 35: Reaching towards the first angle seen from the rear. Arm is soft, left sit bone is light.

As you bring these details into your awareness, also bring your attention to the breath and the jaw to release any unnecessary tension, and pay attention especially to your right arm and shoulder.

Trouble Shooting: 'finishing off'

Quite often what a student will do when they first explore this movement is they will try and **'finish off'** the movement by unnecessarily contracting the shoulder or pectoral muscles. Something that Feldenkrais would have called an unnecessary and 'parasitic' movement (Images 36 and 37).

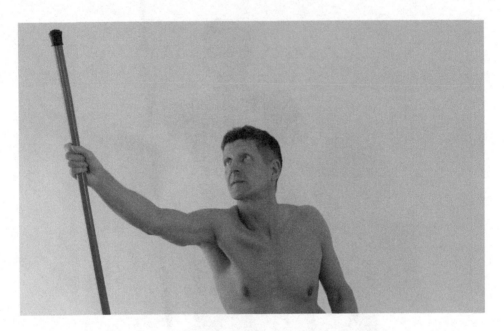

Image 36: An example of 'finishing off'. I've taken my shirt off for this picture so that you can see what I mean by 'finishing off'. Notice how the pectoral muscles around my right collar bone are contracted and compare this with the image below. The movement of the arm and the stick forward should come from the movement of the spine. There is no need to add the redundant pull of the pectoral muscles.

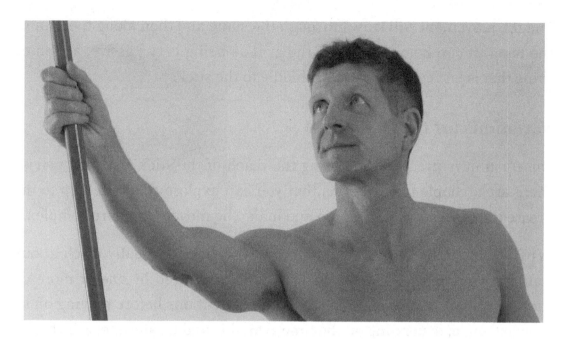

Image 37: Reaching without the 'finishing off'. Notice that my right arm is long but 'soft'. I am not locking out the elbow.

The really important thing to notice, however, is that the reaching of the stick has something to do with the pelvis and the lifting of the left-hand side of the pelvis.

This is a great example of you introducing a **distal-to-core movement**. If you reach the stick far enough, eventually the pelvis will respond. It will be pulled along with the movement. What we now want to do is reverse this pattern to **a core-to-distal** one.

So, now that you have become aware of the role the pelvis can play in reaching the arm and stick, for the next few repetitions see if you can initiate the reaching of the stick by lifting the left side of the pelvis, and the coming back of the stick by lowering the left side of the pelvis.

To an outside observer, this movement will look almost the same, but your internal sense of the movement will be very different indeed. Instead of the movement starting or being initiated from the hand on the stick pulling the spine along, this time you will be initiating the movement from the pelvis and the movement will travel through the spine and then along the arm to the hand. It can help to think of the arm as being very passive, as something that is just connecting your middle to the stick.

Variations for the first angle

Once you have practised initiating the reach of the stick from the pelvis, there are a couple of variations that you can explore that will help to increase the mobility of your spine and make the movement more complex.

When teaching these movements to my students, I typically teach about four or five repetitions of the basic exercise, followed by one or more of these variations with a similar number of repetitions before moving on to the next angle, depending on the time available and whatever else is the focus of the lesson. If you are still starting out on your explorations, feel free to leave the variations out and move on to the next angle (Exercise 10) and come back to these when you are ready.

Exercise 9 Variation A: Turning the head to the left as you reach on diagonal to right

In this variation you reach the stick on the right diagonal as before, initiating from the pelvis, and as you do so, turn the head and eyes to look to the left (Image 38).

As you return to the start position, initiating the return from the pelvis, bring the head and eyes to look forward.

Notice, as you explore this, how far you can **easily** look to the left and pay attention to the difference in the ribs and the shape of your spine that occurs when you turn the head this way.

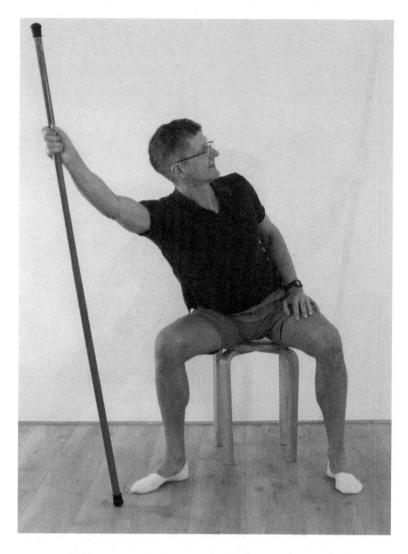

Image 38: Exercise 9A. Looking to the left as I reach the stick forward.

Exercise 9 Variation B: Reaching and turning the head to the right

In this variation, you look to the right with the head and eyes as you reach the stick forward on the first angle, and then look forward again as you bring the stick back (Image 39). It's as if you are looking over your right shoulder but still try to keep your eyes scanning your horizon.

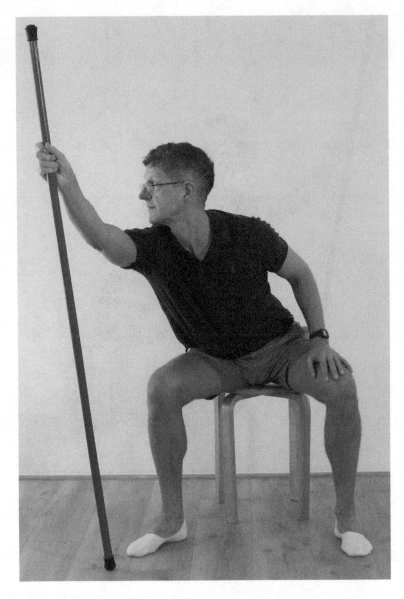

*Image 39: Exercise 9B. Turning the head to the
right as I reach to the first angle.*

Notice how very different this feels to variation A. Does it feel more difficult to look this way? This movement asks for a very different use of the
ribs as we are introducing a more complex twist into the spine. Can you
feel the twist?

Exercise 9 Variation C: Reaching and looking once to the left and then once to the right

In this variation you are looking once to the left and then once to the right as you reach the stick on the diagonal. This gives you a perfect opportunity to test and compare which direction seems 'easier'. Why is that, do you think? What is the spine doing differently? As with all these variations, although you don't need to do too many repetitions, don't rush them because they provide a perfect opportunity to explore how you are moving on any particular day.

Exercise 10: Reaching on the diagonal—second angle (crossing the midline)

One of the most important development milestones is passed when an infant learns to cross their midline, the line that divides them from front to back and helps to establish a left and right side. It remains an important milestone for adults too and requires a great deal of flexibility in the spine and ribs.

Hold the stick in the **right** hand, but this time place the bottom of the stick on the floor in front of the **left** knee and foot. In terms of our clock, the direction of reach is somewhere between 10 and 11 o'clock (Figure I).

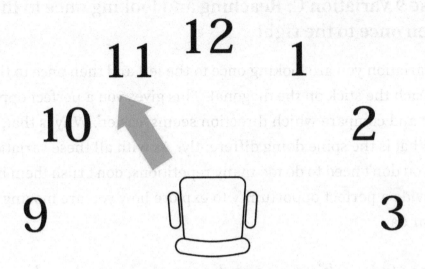

Figure I: Second angle.

Reach the stick away and then back on the left diagonal a few times (Image 40). Look up at the top of the stick as you reach forward, and then look on the horizon as you return. The spine will follow the head and eyes and by looking up it will help to lengthen the front of the body. It's important that you keep the tip of your nose lined up with the stick.

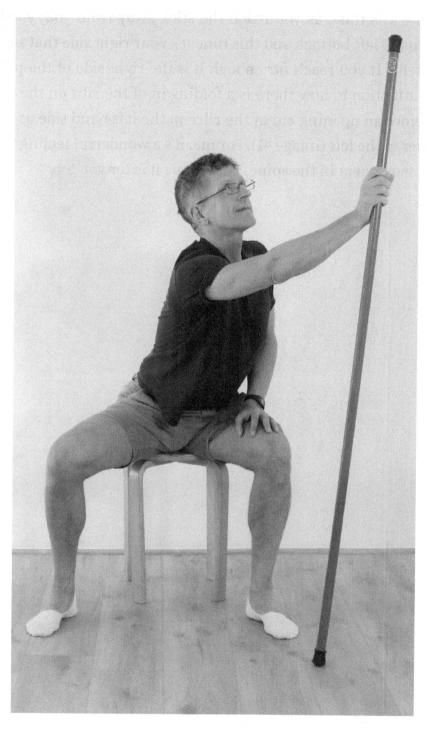

Image 40: Reaching on the second angle. Here my weight has shifted to the left and my right buttock is light. Looking up as you reach the stick will help to lengthen the front of the body.

Notice how this time, as you reach the stick away from you, your weight shifts onto the left buttock and this time it's your right side that side-bends and shortens. If you reach far enough it is the right side of the pelvis that lifts. Pay attention to how there is a folding in of the ribs on the right side and therefore an opening out of the ribs on the left-hand side as the spine curves over to the left (Image 41). For me, it's a wonderful feeling to experience that movement in the spine, and I hope it is for you too.

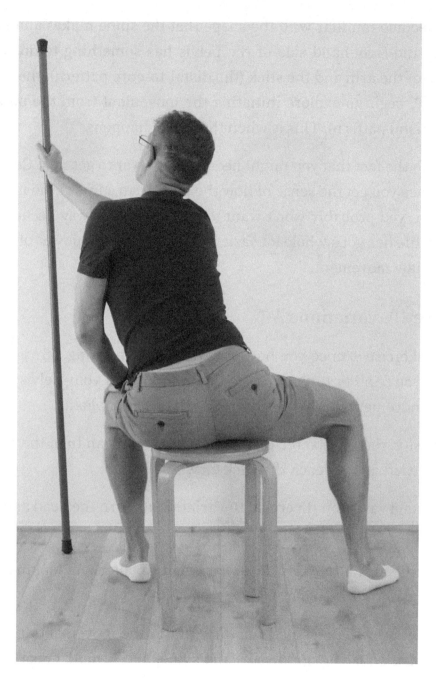

Image 41: Reaching on the diagonal towards the second angle with the stick in my right hand. Viewed from behind, you can clearly see how my weight has transferred onto the left buttock and that the right has become light.

As you become familiar with the shape that the spine makes and how the lifting of the right-hand side of the pelvis has something to do with the reaching of the arm and the stick (the **distal-to-core** pattern), then as with Exercise 9, begin to explore initiating the movement from the pelvis (the **core-to-distal** pattern). This is when the magic happens.

Be open to the fact that you might need to go slower to get this. Certainly, I do, but once you get the sense of how the pelvis can support the movement of the arm you probably won't want to do it any other way because it just feels like life has got a whole lot easier when you use the power of your pelvis to initiate movement.

Exercise 10: Variations A-C

As with Exercise 9, once you have practised this reaching across the midline and your ability to initiate the movement from your pelvis, you can take the movement further by introducing more complexity.

In the first variation (**Exercise 10 Variation A**), you can turn the head and eyes to the left as you reach the stick forward.

In the second variation (**Exercise 10 Variation B**), turn the head and eyes to the right for several repetitions.

In the third variation (**Exercise 10 Variation C**), alternate looking once to the left and once to the right.

Each variation will do something different to the movement and the demands you are placing on the ribs and spine, and I would encourage you, as before, to take the variations slowly so that you can explore and become curious about these differences. You may find, for example, that turning the head in one direction is much easier than the other.

That's great because it means you have information that you can act on as you explore why those differences are there. It might be that in one direction you are more inclined to hold the breath or do something strange with your tongue and jaw that perhaps is unnecessary. These movements become so much more interesting when you approach them like a detective rather than treating them as something just to be got through.

In Exercise 11 we will look at reaching along the midline itself. It's a favourite of mine because something very interesting, as you will discover, happens to the spine.

Exercise 11: Reaching along the midline—third angle

Hold the stick in your right hand as comfortably high up the stick as you can manage without putting strain into your shoulder and line up the stick exactly with your midline i.e., your pubic bone, your navel, your breastbone, the tip of your chin, and your nose. The bottom of the stick should not be too close to you. If I was sitting directly in front of you, I should not be able to see the tip of your nose because your nose would be obscured by the line of the stick (Image 42).

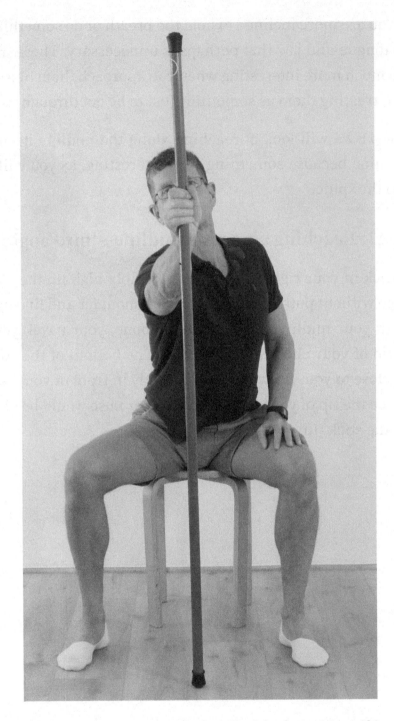

Image 42: Midline reaching towards the 12 o'clock position. If I was sitting directly opposite you as you reach the stick forwards, I should not be able to see the tip of your nose which is lined up with the stick and your hand.

Reach the stick forwards towards the 12 o'clock position and, as before, make sure that every time you reach the stick forwards you look up towards the top of the stick—or, if that is difficult for you, look above the hand that is on the stick (Figure J). As you return to the start position, allow the head and eyes to lower to the horizon.

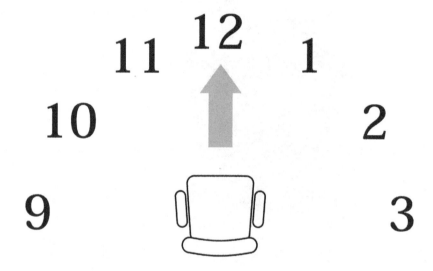

Fig J: The 12 o'clock midline angle.

If you make sure you are reaching the stick directly forward in line with your midline, you will notice a very deep side-bending of the spine over to the left as your weight shifts on to the left sit bone. The right side of your pelvis will become light. The right shoulder and the right side of the pelvis come closer together (Image 43).

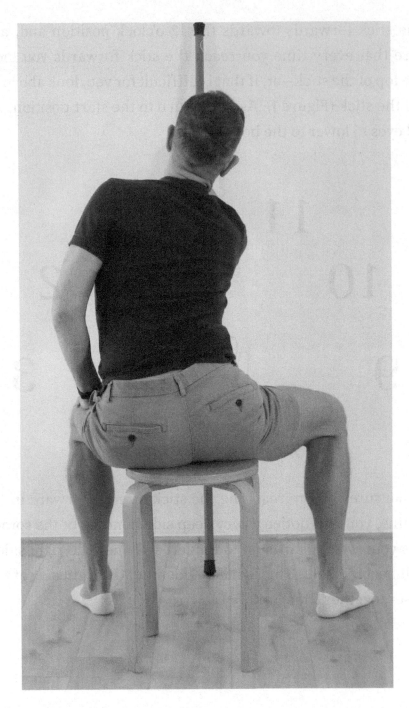

Image 43: Reaching to 12 o'clock viewed from rear. Notice how my weight has shifted over to the left and how my right shoulder is lower than the left. The whole of the right side is shorter than the left, meaning that there is a deep curving of the spine to the left.

Be very fussy about keeping the tip of your nose lined up with the stick as it moves forward. If you are not attentive to this, one of two things will most likely happen if you are currently less mobile in the spine.

The first is that you will begin to move the stick forward and off to the side in an attempt to avoid the movement in the ribs (Image 44 below). The second is that you will move your head to the right or left of the stick as it goes forward, also in an attempt to avoid the side-bending movement (Image 45 below).

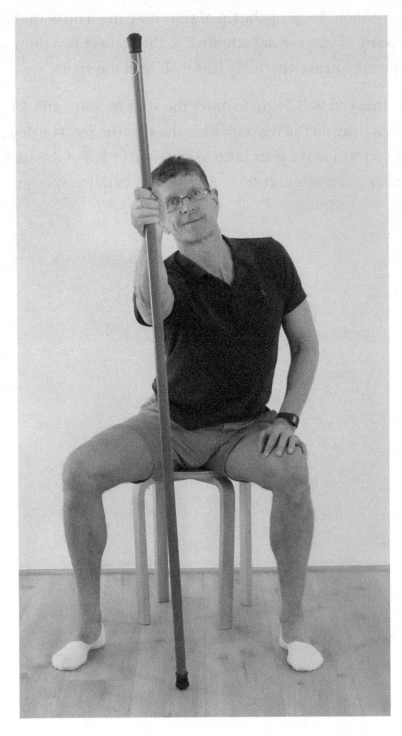

Image 44: Moving the stick to one side to avoid the side-bending.

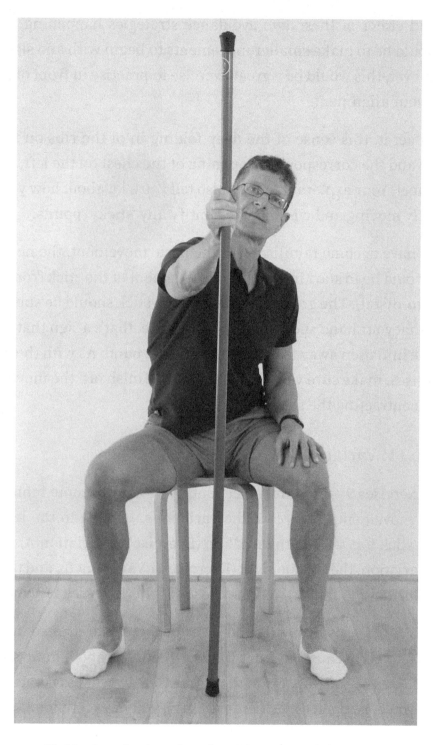

Image 45: Moving the head to the side to avoid the side-bending.

If you find either of these two avoidance strategies happening, then my advice would be to make smaller movements to begin with and slow things down. As ever, this would be a great exercise to practise in front of a mirror to check your alignment.

Once you get it, this sense of the deep folding in of the ribs on the right-hand side and the corresponding opening of the chest on the left, it is wonderful to feel. Your explorations will also tell you a lot about how your spine is currently moving and will help to identify any 'sticky' points.

After you have become familiar with the basic movement, the next step to refine it would be to start initiating the movement of the stick from the pelvis (**core-to-distal**). The grip of the hand on the stick should be super soft. If you find that your hand suddenly becomes tense, that's a sign that you have shifted the initiation away from the pelvis to the hand. As with the previous two exercises, make sure you are not trying to 'finish off' the movement by lifting or contracting the shoulder.

Exercise 11: Variations A-C

As with Exercises 9 and 10, feel free, once you have become familiar with the main movement, to explore the variations: looking to the left as you reach the stick forward on the midline (**Exercise 11 Variation A**) would be the first variation, then to the right (**Exercise 11 Variation B**), and then alternate looking once to the left and then to the right (**Exercise 11 Variation C**).

If you have a scoliosis, you will find some of these exercises so interesting and useful to do because of what they will tell you about your spine and how it is currently moving. From that increased awareness comes choices, and once you have choices, Feldenkrais said, you have freedom.

The other side and a pep talk!

If you haven't already done so as you have been exploring the exercises in Chapters 1 and 2, now would be a very good time to repeat Exercises 1 to 11 but with the stick in the left hand.

You would start with the exercises in Chapter 1 with side-bending to the left and then move on to the exercises and variations in Chapter 2. As you explore the use of the left side, be open to the fact that there may be very real differences between how this side is moving compared to the right. Don't try and muscle through these differences or pretend that they are not there. Such differences are important information for you to explore and act upon and can tell you a lot about any habits and holding patterns that you may have.

I realise in writing the former paragraph that it can sound frustratingly zen-like and obscure. I don't mean it to be. I am rather embarrassed to say that when I first started this work after my own injury, I approached it with the mindset of a lawyer who was used to cross-examining witnesses and getting answers to my questions (I was a barrister specialising in criminal law). I had this constant mindset that I wanted to get things 'right', but sometimes there is no 'one answer' and no 'one way of doing it'. It is your own answer and your own way of doing it that is important, not somebody else's. It took me a long time to realise that this rather anal lawyer's mindset was actually getting in the way of progress.

There is no one right way of moving or one final goal to achieve because we are all different and we are individually different from one day to the next.

Sometimes you might be dealing with an injury, emotional or physical. You might not have had enough sleep the night before and therefore your system will be off.

Your guide to change is to look for what is easy and effortless. The moments when your breath is easy and when you are free of unnecessary tension, whether that be in the jaw or elsewhere. The range of easy movement may be very small on one day, but if you confine yourself to what is easy and stay within that boundary then progress will come because it's only when your nervous system does not feel under threat that it will be open to doing something different. It's often our ego that gets in the way of that. You may feel, as I often did, deflated by the fact that there is something you can't do easily today, but acceptance of that fact opens the door to the possibility that you may do it differently tomorrow. Be kind to yourself in your practice.

Summary

By the time you have explored the exercises in this chapter you will have gained a very deep, embodied understanding of how you can support the movement of your arms from your spine and pelvis. We have used the stick to bring that possibility back 'online'.

To return to the car analogy I introduced at the beginning of the chapter, if you have followed the exercises, you will have effectively jump-started the engine back into life as you learnt how to integrate the movement of the pelvis into the use of your arms to reach. But we don't want this learning to be confined to the time you are doing your exercises. We would like that learning to carry over into your day-to-day life.

The next time you reach for something at your kitchen table, at your desk, or in a supermarket, see if you can begin to change the way that you think about how you are reaching to include the pelvis and the spine. You may feel a little self-conscious to begin with, but it will knock years off your 'movement age' and will help keep your spine young and mobile.

We will return to this reaching movement when we look at coming to stand in Chapter 6 Exercises 18 and 19.

In the next chapter, we will be looking at another two very important movements of your spine: the ability to flex and extend it. We will also consider how this ability can support your posture, balance, and so much more besides.

3 / FLEXION AND EXTENSION

On my YouTube channel I have a mat-based Feldenkrais lesson called *'Fabulous Flexors: How to Improve your Abdominals the Feldenkrais Way'*. I first uploaded it in 2018 and when I could be bothered to look at what's called the 'analytics', I discovered with interest that this video was, for a time, watched by proportionally more men than women compared to all my other videos. I am not sure what inferences I should draw from that interesting nugget of data, but what I do know is that, putting the aesthetics of the elusive six-pack to one side, your abdominal and back muscles play a vital role in your ability to move well.

In broad terms that are sufficient for our purposes, your muscles can be divided into two groups: your flexors and your extensors.

Flexors are the muscles that help to close the angle or space between your joints and bones. When you bend your arm, your bicep muscles act as the flexors of the elbow.

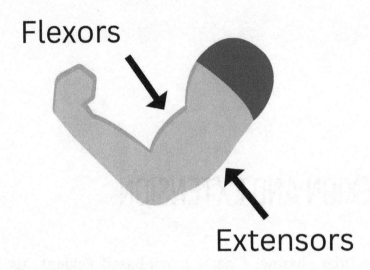

Figure K: An example of flexors and extensors.

Your extensors are the muscles that open the angle or space between your bones. When you straighten your arm, your triceps extend your elbow.

When you curl up into a ball you are using your flexors. When you lie on your front and lift your head, arms and legs off the floor, you are primarily using your extensors.

Your abdominal muscles can therefore be considered as part of your flexors. Your back muscles are part of your extensors.

Functionally though, your back and stomach muscles do so much more than simply bend and straighten you. They play a part in your ability to breathe, make love, digest, excrete, move, balance, stand, walk, run and so much more besides. The ability to use your flexors and extensors well, in a way that supports your day-to-day life and needs, is vital to the question of how well you as a boomer will age. Let's look at two examples of what I mean: vision and standing.

Functional vision

We tend to think of vision as something that simply concerns the eyes. Certainly, the acuity and health of your eyes is part of the equation, but if you are lucky enough to work, as I do, with children with needs, you quickly learn that we don't just see with the eyes but also with the brain. Even if the eyes are healthy, damage to the brain can result in significant impairment of vision.

Beyond the question of your actual ability to see and process images, however, your functional vision has something to do with your ability to move well. So, what do I mean here by functional vision?

As human beings we are unique in the animal world in that we are the only creatures who have evolved to organise our movement around a vertical axis. You have two eyes and two ears located in your head at the top of your spine. You have this ability to turn around your vertical axis to position your eyes and ears and nose (known as 'teleceptors') towards an object or sound on the horizon, and this gives us important information that we can act upon. Our brain processes differences between the data coming from the right and left eyes and ears to tell us all sorts of things about what is in the space around us and how we are positioned in relation to that space.

In former times, this might have been vital information about how near or far a threat to our safety was located or where prospective food was escaping. In more immediately relevant circumstances, it might be information about how fast a car is approaching as you are trying to cross a road while your arms are busy with shopping or a child. Our two eyes and ears are forward facing, and being able to turn them towards the threat or target is a vital skill.

Quite often you will see a person whose flexors and extensors are not well organised. The back is rounded, the neck is short and tight. When this person tries to look about themselves, their ability to look is severely compromised because their spine is 'busy' with these holding patterns. This compromised functional vision can make an elderly person very vulnerable. If they can't see something coming, they are unlikely to know that they need to avoid a possible threat to their balance (Image 46).

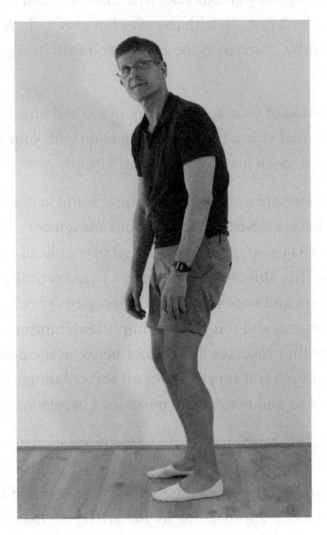

Image 46: In this image you can see that my back is rounded, my pelvis is tucked under, and my knees are bent. My head has come forward and, if you look closely, you will see that my head is now located in the space above my toes. Because I am overworking my flexors, I am now not able to organise around the vertical axis of my spine. This means that when I turn to look at something, most of that movement is coming from the upper part of the neck, and as a result there is a part of the world around me that I cannot easily see: the area behind me.

A person, however, who is able to organise around a long vertical spine has a much better chance, should the issue arise, of seeing an impending threat approaching and therefore of taking avoiding action (Image 47).

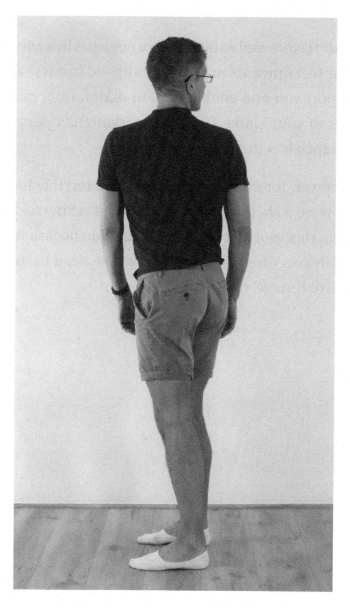

Image 47: In this image my legs are straight without being locked, my head is floating on top of my spine and most of my weight is passing through my skeleton into my heels. My flexors and extensors are much more balanced and therefore I am able to turn around my vertical axis to see all the way around myself.

You can therefore appreciate how a more skilful use of your flexors and extensors can support your functional vision.

Standing

In standing, your flexors and extensors are engaged in a constant spiralling dance from your feet upwards to keep you aligned in a way that allows your skeleton to support you and enables you to maintain organisation around the vertical axis of your spine. Quite often, though, a person's posture reveals that this dance has turned into a collapse.

When I was a lawyer, for example, I developed a terrible habit of using my stomach as if it were a shelf upon which I could rest my folded arms. Quite a lot of people do this, not just lawyers. Fine to do occasionally, I suppose, but repeated daily can often, and did in my case, lead to something called sway back posture (Image 48).

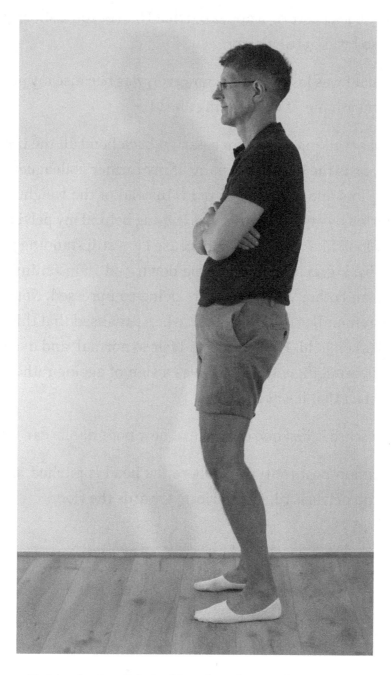

Image 48: I had a terrible habit, when I was a lawyer, of using my stomach as if it were a shelf to rest my folded arms on. Over time, this 'sway back' posture became my norm. I used to suffer from back pain all the time and was constantly visiting physios or osteopaths to get it sorted but always returned because the fundamental cause, my poor organisation, hadn't been addressed. The thing is, I had no idea that I was doing this, walking around with my pelvis leading.

With my sway back posture, it appeared that I had become shorter. I thought it was because I was getting older.

The reason that I was losing height, however, was because my pelvis was no longer underneath me. It was trailing ahead.

In effect, I was walking around in a partial back bend all the time and, not surprisingly, as is the case with many of my former colleagues at the Bar, I was getting lots and lots of back pain. Instead of the weight of my head being supported by my skeleton, it was lagging behind my pelvis. It may not immediately look like a 'fall' to you because I am still standing on two legs, but in sway back gravity is pulling me down and I am falling. My spine, heart, lungs, and other vital organs are being compressed. Not a good look really. I can remember the shock I felt when I realised that this sway back posture had taken hold. Everything had felt so normal, and like many people I rather begrudgingly thought it was a sign of ageing rather than waking up to the fact that it was a habit.

Sway back posture is just one example of how poor habits can take hold.

Another common posture-type is where the head is pitched forward, and the front of the pelvis is tilted anteriorly towards the floor.

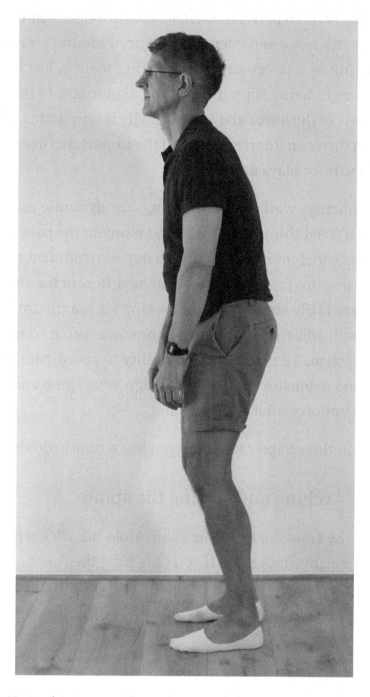

Image 49: In this image I have let my abdominals go and my pelvis is tilted forwards—the anterior tilt. You can see that my weight has shifted to the front of my feet and as my spine is now 'falling again' I am having to shorten the back of my neck to keep my head and eyes on the horizon. Often, when I work with a client with this postural habit, they have very collapsed arches in the front of the feet.

With an anteriorly tilted pelvis the flexors are no longer helping to hug your organs against the spine and keep you balanced around a vertical axis but are simply acting as a safety net. Vertical alignment is lost and instead of the person's weight being supported by the diaphragm of the pelvic floor, the anterior part of the lower abdominal cavity is now acting as a poor substitute. This in turn can interfere with all the important functions in which a healthy pelvic floor plays a part.

Standing, balancing, walking, and sitting are dynamic activities. Good posture is not a fixed thing but a place and moment in space and time that depends on our constant interaction with our environment and ourselves. What is 'good' posture for one activity will be different for another, but the ground rules are fairly simple. We are looking for maximum support from our skeleton with adjustments to our alignment coming from our muscles and nervous system. That requires the ability to coordinate the actions of your flexors and extensors to be able to align your spine and pelvis in the way that best supports what you are doing.

The exercises in this chapter will help you learn how to do that.

Exercise 12: Arching and curling the spine

Come to sit at the front edge of your chair. Hold the stick with both hands at about chest height (Image 50). If you only have the functional use of one arm, then all the exercises in this chapter can be done using a single arm.

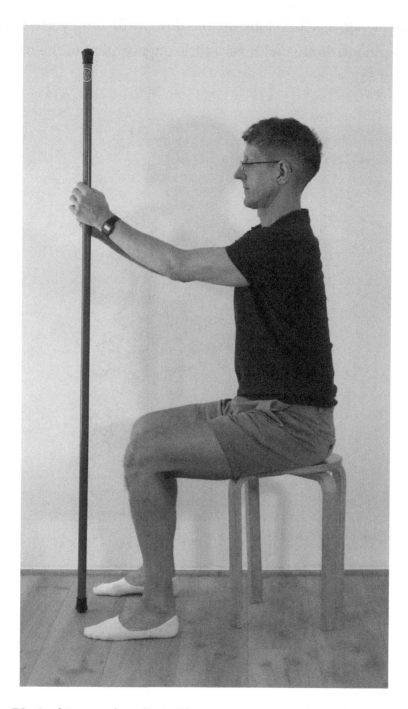

Image 50: Arching and curling. The start position viewed from the side.

The instructions are simple: look up at the top of the stick and then look down at the bottom of the stick. However, it's what you do to look up and down that is important.

Many people when asked to look up and down will simply use the cervical part of the spine to do this with very little engagement of the back and the pelvis (Image 51).

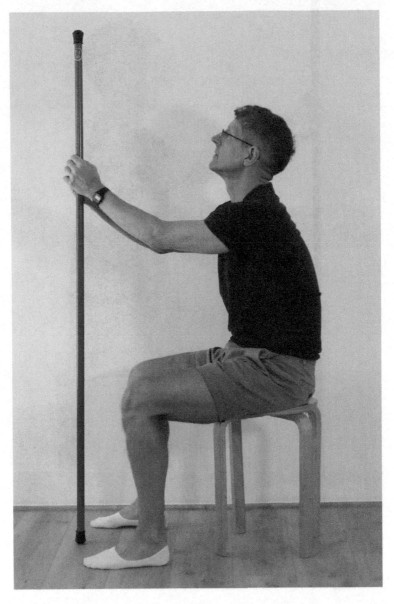

Image 51: In this image you can see that I am looking up but only using the very upper part of my neck. You can see the folds in my skin above the collar of my clothing at the back. The rest of my spine is completely rounded. Instead of my spine having four curves, it now has only two. You will see this often when a person is sitting at a desk working at their computer. The spine has collapsed, and all the strain is taken by the neck.

What we are looking for, however, is a global or integrated use of the spine.

So, from the start position, when you look down at the bottom of the stick see if you can round the whole of the spine. This requires you to soften the chest, pull the ribs in and down, and at the same time pull in your tummy (Image 52).

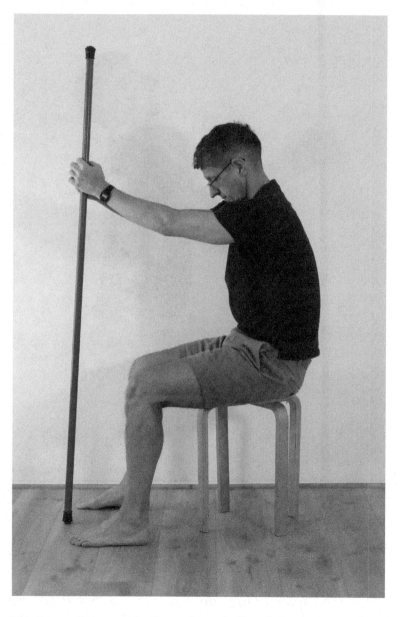

Image 52: Rounding, or curling, the whole of the spine to look down.

When you look up at the top of the stick, arch the spine and think of lengthening the breastbone and the pubic bone away from each other, pushing out the lower tummy (Image 53).

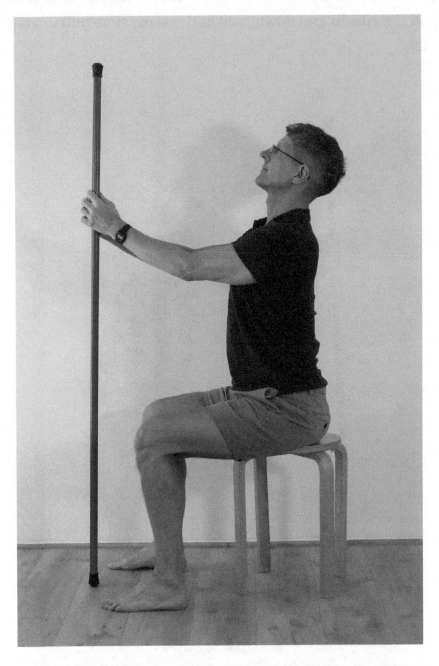

Image 53: Arching the spine to look up. You can see that there are no creases now in the back on the neck because the whole of the spine is engaged.

You will find it easier to breathe out as you round the back to look down and to breathe in as you lengthen the front of the spine and look up.

As you explore arching and curling the spine in this way, the important thing to remember is this: imagine in your mind's eye that there is a vertical line drawn to your side that connects the outer shoulder to the outer hip.

As you round the back, keep the outer shoulder stacked over the outer hip (Image 54).

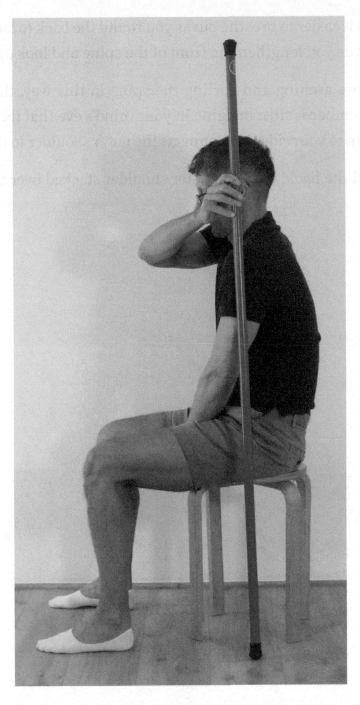

Image 54: I need an extra pair of hands! The idea here is that you imagine that there is a vertical line connecting your outer shoulder to your outer hip so that when you round the back to look down, you keep the shoulder positioned vertically in space over the hip and avoid displacing the upper body forward and back.

As you arch the back, also keep the outer shoulder aligned over the hip (Image 55).

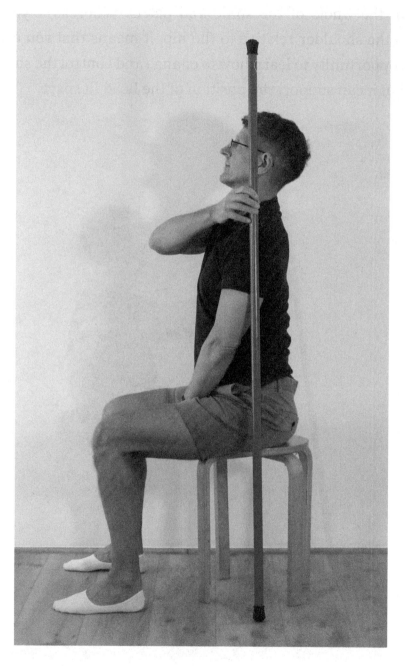

Image 55: As you arch the back to look up, keep the outer shoulder stacked above the outer hip.

If you can do this, and it will require some practice and honest feedback from a mirror or friend, then it means you are asking the movement to come from the whole of the spine and pelvis. Whereas if you **displace** (Image 56) the shoulder relative to the hip, it means that you are missing out on the opportunity to learn how to change and control the shape of your spine so that it can support the position of the head in space.

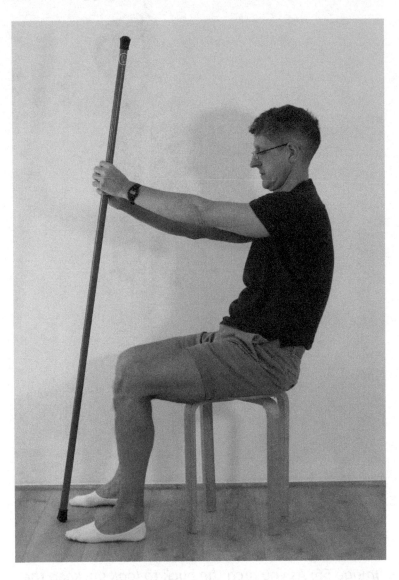

Image 56: This is an example of what I mean by 'displacing'. Here, I have simply leant backwards to look down and moved my upper body behind my pelvis. Sure, this will help me to look down, but there is no real change in the spine.

Practise this arching and curling with the stick until you become familiar with the shape of the spine that we are looking for. Don't be too hard on yourself if it feels a bit clunky to begin with. It will improve with practice for sure.

Once you have had a little practice, here are two pointers to think about that will help you to refine the movement.

The feet

The first pointer is to pay attention to what is happening to the feet. If you bring your awareness to the feet as you are rounding and arching the spine, you will notice something very interesting.

As you are rounding the back, it's as if the feet want to push forward, and as you are rounding the back it's as if the feet want to drag backwards on the floor.

This happens because of the connection of your leg muscles to the pelvis and the shift of weight to the back and front of your sit bones. So, let's use this tendency to actively help with the arching and curling.

Don't move the feet at all but as you round the back to look down at the floor think of pushing forward through the feet, but don't move them (Image 57).

Then as your arch the back, again without moving the feet, think of dragging the feet and floor back towards you (Image 58).

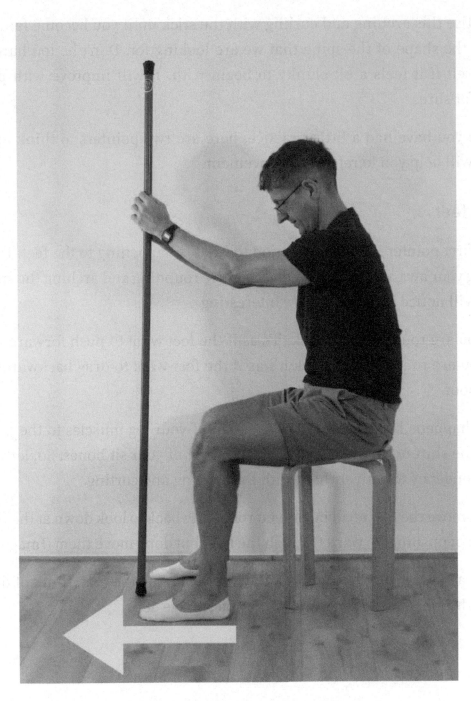

Image 57: As you round the back, push the feet forwards without moving them.

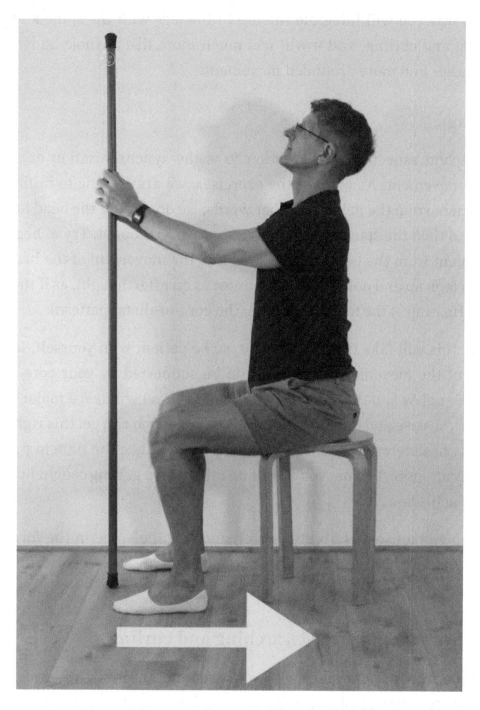

*Image 58: As you arch the back, drag the feet
backwards without moving them.*

In this way you will integrate the use of the legs with the spine and your arching and curling, and it will feel much more like a whole body event, with easier and more grounded movement.

Timing

The second aspect to pay attention to is the synchronisation or timing of the movement. As with all the exercises, we are looking to initiate the movement from the pelvis. In other words, we don't want the head to move first and then the spine and the pelvis as an afterthought. Try to begin the movement from the pelvis upwards so that the movement of the head and eyes to look up and down happens almost as an afterthought, as if the head is just floating at the top of the spine (the **core-to-distal** pattern).

Again, this will take time to get right, so be patient with yourself. Ideally, we want the movement of the head to be supported by your core rather than the pelvis and the spine playing catch-up. You will feel a major difference in the ease and quality of your movement if you can get this right, and there's absolutely no reason why you can't if you take the time to practise and pay attention to what you are doing rather than getting caught up in the idea of achievement.

Let's now practise this ability to arch and flex the spine in the form of a more dynamic movement that feels fantastic for any of you suffering from an achy back.

Exercise 13: Spinal waves arching and curling

Sit at the front of your chair with your feet and knees slightly wider than hip distance apart. Hold the stick with both hands at a height that is level with the top of your breastbone.

Arch the back and look at the top of the stick, paying attention to all the teaching points from the previous exercise.

Once you have come into your spinal arch, stay arched and then reach the stick forward until you can't reach any further. Your arms remain straight but not locked (Image 59).

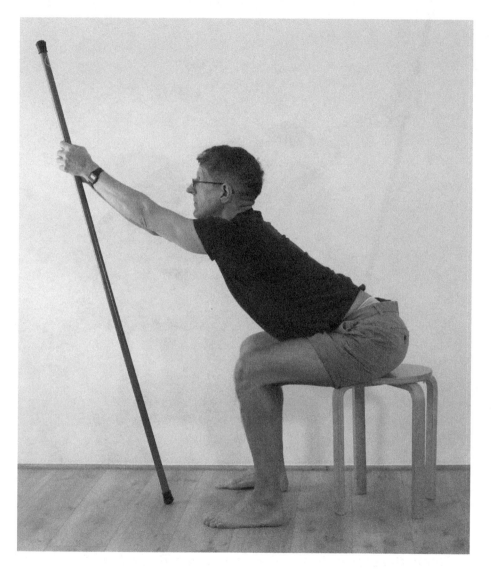

Image 59: Reaching as far forward as I can in the arched position.

Once you have reached forward, release the head, and bring your ears between your upper arms so that you are now looking down at the floor (Image 60).

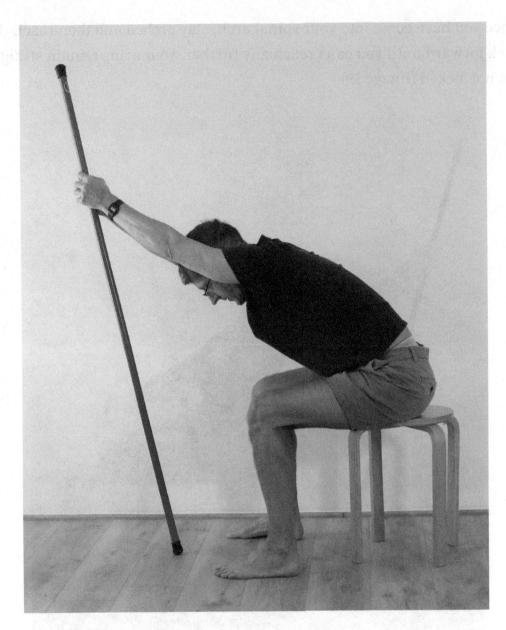

Image 60: Once you have reached forward in the arch, look down and bring the ears between the upper arms. Begin to push forward through the feet, pull in the tummy and begin to curl back.

Begin to curl back from the pelvis by pulling in the lower abdomen, softening the chest, and pushing forward through the feet to curl yourself back onto the chair—the head is the last thing to arrive (Image 61).

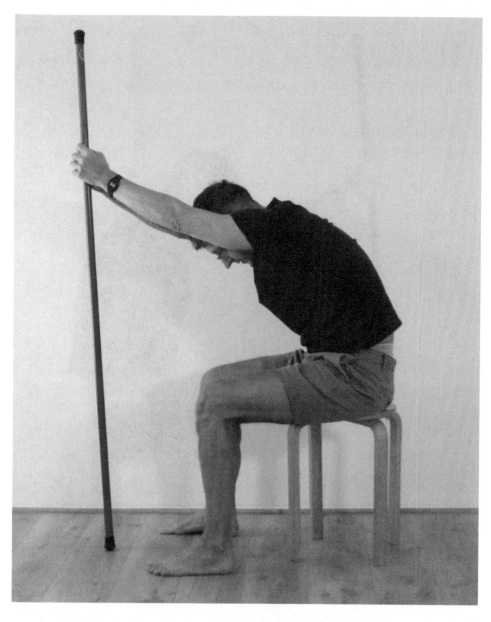

Image 61: Here I am curling back from the pelvis, allowing the head to linger.

Once you arrive back on the chair in your curled position (Image 62), with the outer shoulders stacked over the outer hips, release into the neutral start position, neither arched nor curled, and then you can begin to arch again and repeat the sequence several times.

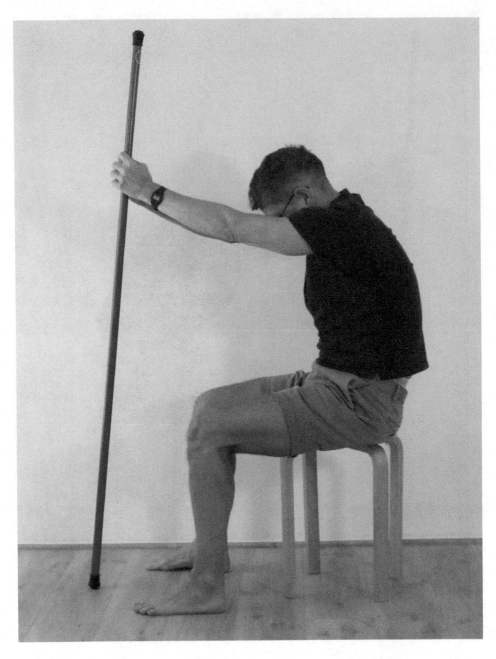

Image 62: Arriving back on the chair in the curled position, ready to release into neutral and then into the arch to repeat the sequence.

Five or six repetitions should do the trick, but the movement feels so nice you will probably want to do more. As you become familiar with the sequence you will be able to flow from one arch and curl into the next.

The key point to pay attention to is that you are not lifting the head too early. If you do lift it too early, it will cause back muscles to contract on the return instead of releasing and lengthening as you engage your flexors to come back. Think of the head lingering all the time. You can think of your arms as being completely passive to avoid any unnecessary tension creeping into the shoulders and hands.

In the next exercise, the pattern is simply reversed.

Exercise 14: Spinal waves curl and arch

From your neutral start position, curl your spine, look down, and as you reach forward bring your ears between the upper arms. It's as if you are about to dive into water (Image 63).

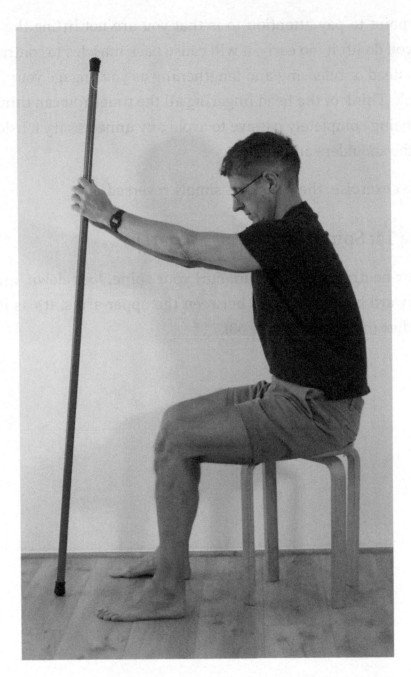

Image 63: From neutral, begin to curl the spine and look down,
pushing forward through the feet, and then reach forward.

Keep the rounded shape of your spine as you reach the stick as far forward as you comfortably can (Images 64 and 65).

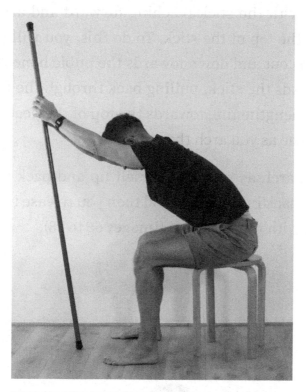

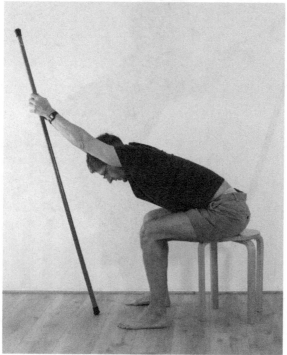

Images 64 and 65: Keep the rounded shape of your spine as you reach forward.

Then stay there with the stick reaching forward and arch the spine and look up towards the top of the stick. To do this, you will need to push the lower abdominals out and down towards the pubic bone and lengthen the breast bone towards the stick, pulling back through the feet. Think of the front of the body lengthening towards the top of the head and towards the tip of your tail bone as you arch the back.

Then stay in the arch as you lift yourself up and back to the seat of the chair. You arrive back in your arch and then you release into neutral before beginning again with the sequence (Images 66 to 68).

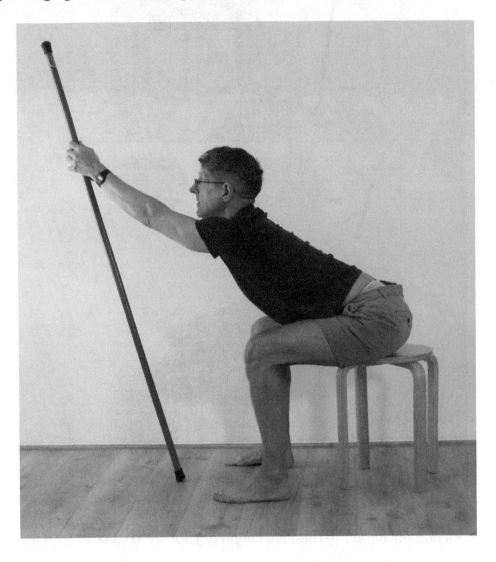

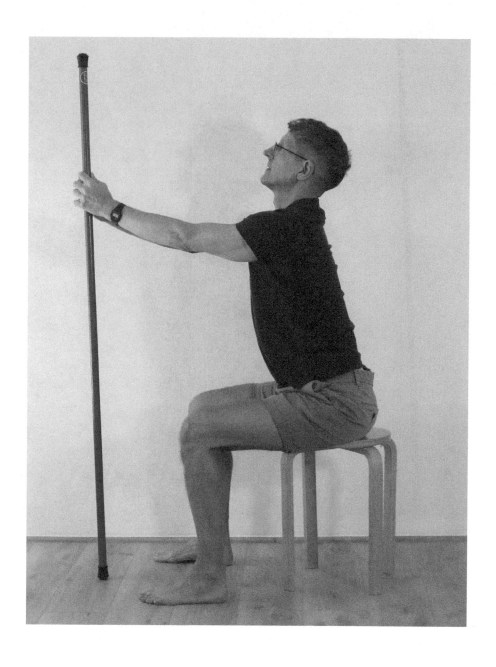

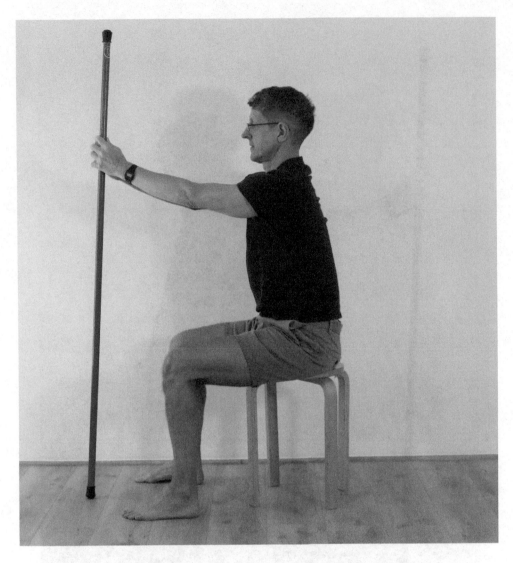

Images 66, 67, and 68: Releasing into the arch, coming back in an arch, and then releasing into neutral, ready to begin curling again.

Final thoughts

Don't be surprised, as you first explore the spinal wave sequences, if you discover that certain parts of your spine are a bit 'sticky'. It will take time for your muscles and ligaments to adapt to the new demands that are being placed on them. Becoming aware of these 'sticky' areas is a good thing because that is the door opening to the possibility of change. When I sense these 'sticky' areas, my strategy, and one that I recommend to you, is to slow things down.

Your nervous system is re-learning refined motor control of segments of your spine that may have been neglected for some years. However, once you discover the possibility of initiating these spinal waves from your centre, it will have a profound impact on your ability to initiate movement in other contexts. One thing that may inspire you to keep your motivation is to look around at people as they go about their daily lives and try to assess how much the person is initiating movement from their centre. Those in trouble with their movement are the ones who aren't. This is not to judge them but to see if you can recognise patterns that you may well share and to learn from them, to refine your own awareness of movement. It's often easier to see these patterns in others rather than to recognise it in yourself. I think of my own 'sway back' posture, for example.

One of the hidden benefits of the spinal wave exercises is that we have also been exploring shifting your weight away from the seat of the chair and into the feet from the core. We will be coming back to this more explicitly in Chapter 6 when we explore coming to stand up effortlessly.

To fully prepare for that part of the programme and to give your arms a bit of a break from all the stick work, now would be a good time to turn our attention to the feet, knees, and hips, and that's what we will do in the next chapter.

4 / FEET, KNEES, AND HIPS

In the West, our environment and daily routines often conspire to constrict the range of movement in our joints, and this is especially the case for our feet, knees, and hips.

The cumulative effect over time of certain kinds of shoes, flat pavements, clothing, work practices, inactive sitting, and norms of social and cultural behaviour is often that muscles around these joints become locked into certain habits and lengths as the nervous system adapts to these impositions.

This movement deficit is no doubt one of the major contributors to the huge number of joint replacement surgeries that take place each year throughout the Western world, a majority of these patients being 50 years old or older, the Baby Boomer generation.

At the other end of the age spectrum, if you look at toddlers on the move, they transition from the floor to their sides, sitting, kneeling, standing, walking, squatting, and back down again almost effortlessly. Their feet, knees and hips don't get in the way of their movement but play a vital role in an infant's ability to weight-transfer from one position to the next (Images 69 to 71).

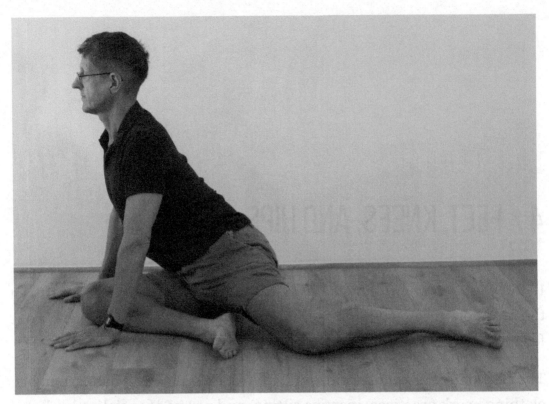

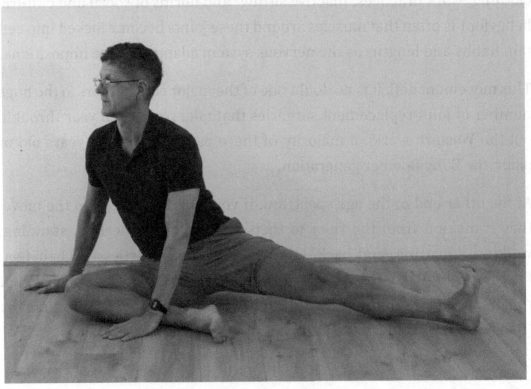

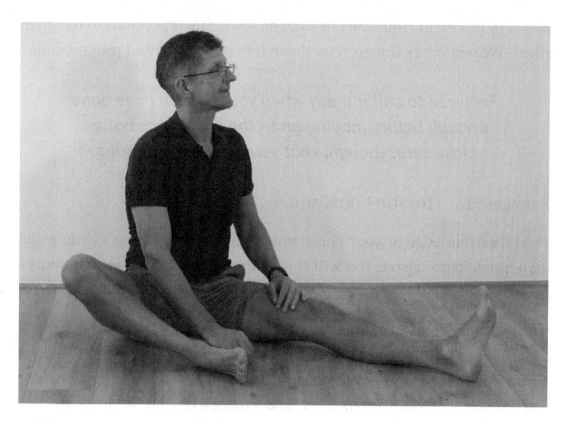

Image 69, 70, 71: I am certainly not a toddler, and I didn't have one conveniently at hand to photograph, but you can see that the flexibility of our hips, knees, and feet play a vital role in our ability to weight-transfer efficiently and transition from one position to another. Often when these joints aren't available to absorb and transmit movement then the 'slack' gets taken up by the back trying to do its best to compensate.

If your feet, knees, and hips are not working as they could do, and you are not using them as you could do to support your movement, then the repercussions of this will be felt in your joints and back, and over time they will adversely affect your mobility and independence. Do you have a knee problem, for example, or is the knee issue a symptom of a movement deficit?

It's time to start looking after your legs, and the exercise in this lesson will help you do that. It simulates the same movement skills that you developed as a toddler. Be warned, though, that while this exercise is simple to do, it is also very powerful. You won't need to do too many repetitions to feel their effect. We will break the exercise down into easily followed progressions.

> *Feel free to call it a day when you feel you have done enough before moving on to the next progression.*
> *Make sure, though, that you explore both sides.*

Exercise 15: The start position

Sit at the front edge of your chair with your feet and knees a little wider than hip distance apart. You will find it helpful for this exercise to wear a pair of socks.

Place one end of the stick so that it rests against the top of your left thigh, somewhere near the groin. The other end of the stick is resting on the floor. If you were sitting at the centre of a clock with 12 o'clock immediately in front of you, 3 o'clock to your right, and 9 o'clock to your left, then the bottom of the stick would be resting somewhere around the 2 o'clock position. The hands are taking hold lightly towards the top of the stick (Image 72).

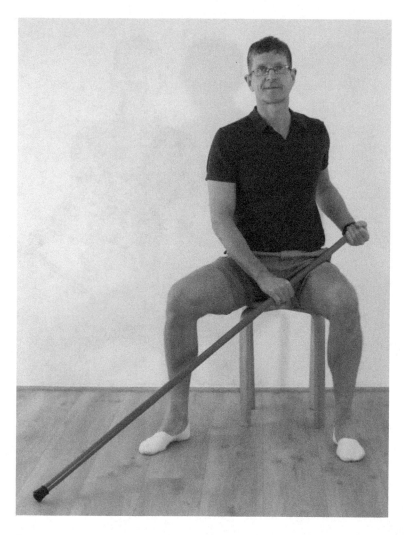

Image 72: The starting position for the hip exercise with the stick at 2 o'clock.

Exercise 15: First progression

The first part of the exercise is simply to see if you can place your right foot on the stick and then take it back off again (Image 73).

Do this several times. Once you have tried this, pause for a moment, rest, and notice how the right hip feels.

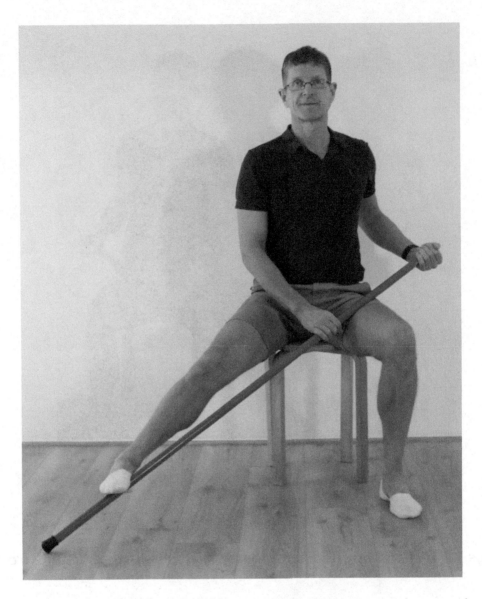

Image 73: Putting my right foot on the stick. Seems simple enough but for many people this is already quite a challenge.

Again, a reminder: for many people this seemingly simple movement can represent a real challenge in and of itself. If you need to leave it at that for today, that's absolutely fine; try it on the other side, move on to the next chapter, and come back to this exercise another day. Be kind to yourself. Otherwise, carry on to the next progression.

Exercise 15: **Second progression**

If you are comfortable resting the right foot on the stick, keep it there for the next progression.

Begin to slide your foot up the stick, and as you do so, turn the sole of the foot towards you as if you wanted to see if there is something stuck on the bottom of your foot. As the foot slides up the stick, allow the right knee to rotate out to the side (Image 74).

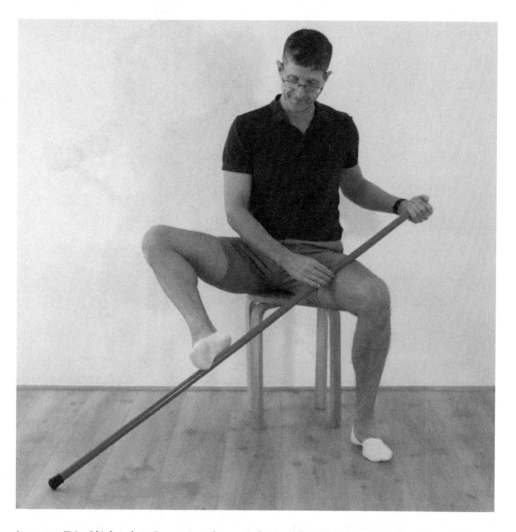

Image 74: Slide the foot up the stick and look at the sole of your foot. Can you see how I am allowing the right knee to rotate out to the side as the foot travels up the stick and also how I have allowed— remembering the previous chapter—my back to round as I look down?

Then slide the foot back down the stick, straightening the leg, turning the sole of the foot away from you, and push the heel away from you so that you are dorsiflexing the foot. It's as if you are using the leg and foot to push or kick something at the end of the foot further away from you (Image 75).

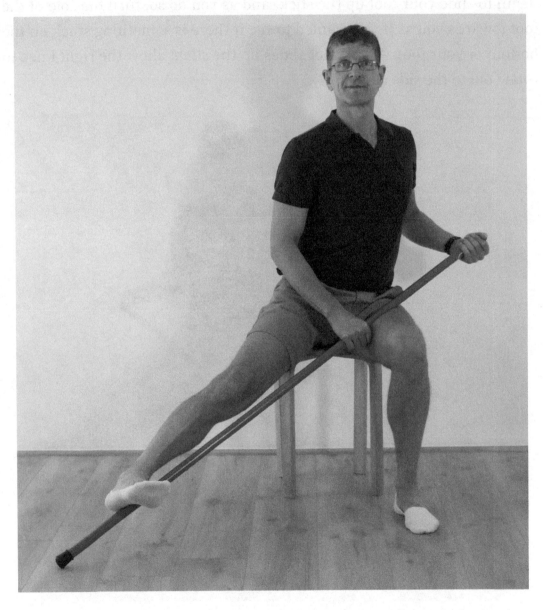

Image 75: As I slide the foot down the stick pushing through the heel and dorsiflex the foot as shown, notice how my weight has shifted more towards my left sit bone and how my spine has lengthened.

To begin with, make this a small movement up and down the stick. You will feel some powerful things happening in the ankle, calf muscles, knees, and hips. Remember to fully push the heel away from you as you straighten the leg and to turn the sole of the foot towards you as you slide it up the stick. In this way you will begin to integrate, or synchronise, the movement of the foot with the knee, hip, and pelvis.

After a few repetitions, take the foot off the stick and notice what you feel in the hips. You can now choose to repeat these instructions on the other leg and call it a day, or if you feel comfortable with this step then proceed directly to the next progression.

Exercise 15: Third progression

You can now begin to explore making a bigger movement up the stick. Go slowly but see how far you can comfortably slide the foot up the stick, turning the sole of the foot towards you, and always fully lengthening the leg and dorsiflexing the foot as it travels away from you.

As you explore this bigger movement something very interesting begins to happen to your pelvis and spine (Images 76 and 77).

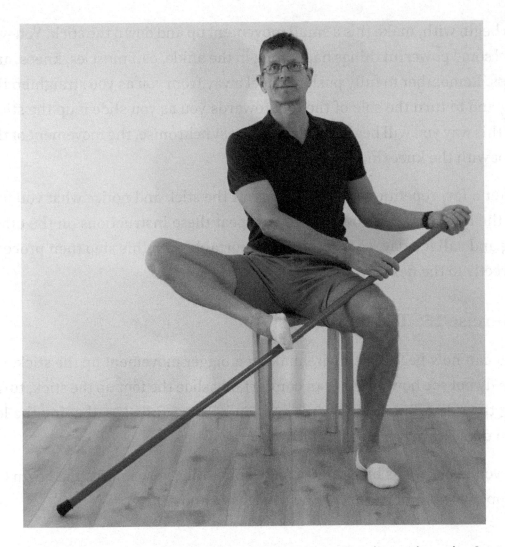

Image 76: As you explore a bigger movement, notice how when the foot comes towards you, your weight tends to shift onto both your sit bones.

When the foot travels up the stick, your weight tends to shift on to your two sit bones, but when you straighten the leg away, your weight tends to shift on to your left sit bone and the pelvis rotates to the left. This sets off a whole chain reaction of movement as the spine spirals and lengthens all the way up to the top of the head. It's the most marvellous feeling of physics-in-action, the sense of an equal and opposite reaction: as the leg moves down and away, the spine spirals up and away on a diagonal and what connects the two directions is of course your pelvis.

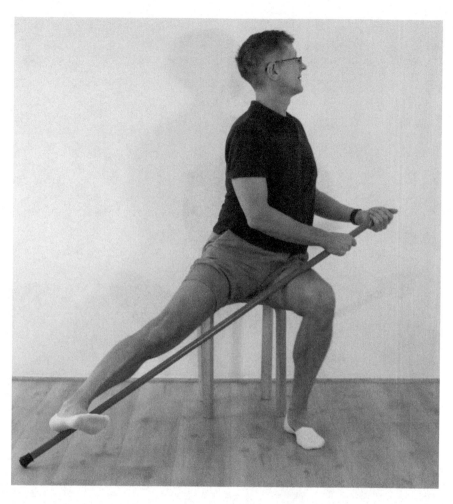

Image 77: If you really focus on lengthening the leg and heel away from you, your weight will shift to the left sit bone and the pelvis rotates to create a lengthening spiral that travels all along the spine to the crown of the head.

Remember this feeling of lengthening down and away from the pelvis to the foot and up and away to the head. This is the same feeling that we will be looking to reproduce in standing. The sense of being very grounded from the pelvis and lengthening in two directions (Images 78 and 79).

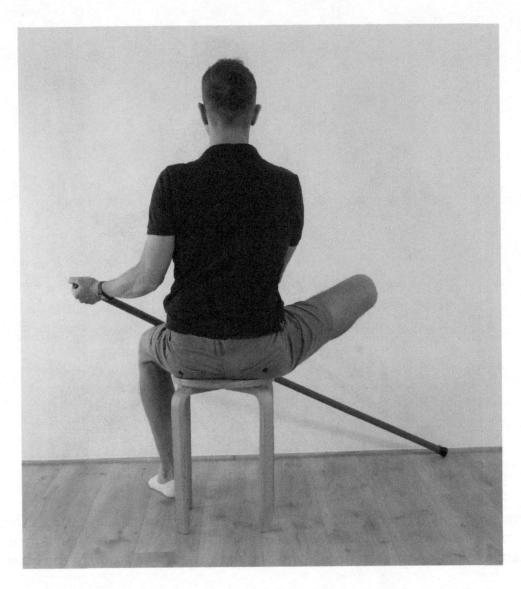

Image 78: It is easier to see the weight shift and the movement of the pelvis from the rear. Notice how my weight is on two sit bones as my foot slides up the stick. Contrast this with the next image.

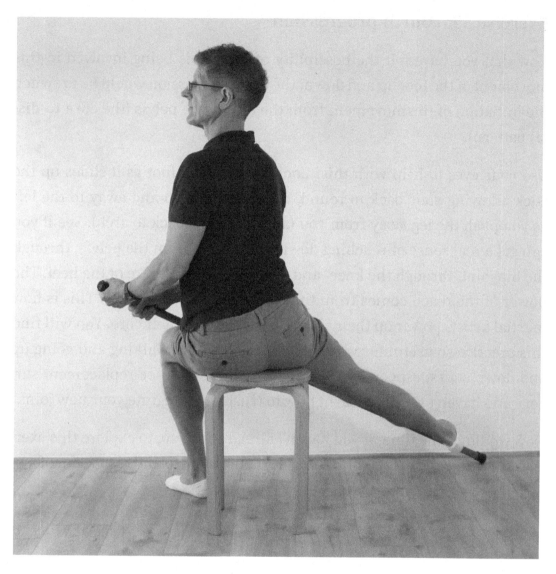

Image 79: Notice how my weight has shifted to my left sit bone as I push my right leg and heel away. It creates this delicious sense of a spiral travelling up through the spine and out of the top of the head. There are two lengthenings radiating from the core: to the foot and to the head.

Exercise 15: **Fourth progression**

Now that you have felt the possibility of the pelvis being involved in this movement of the foot up and down, the next progression would be to switch the initiation of the movement from the foot to the pelvis (the **core-to-distal** pattern).

Use your eyes to help with this. Look down at the foot as it slides up the stick allowing your back to round, and then look up and away to the left as you push the leg away from you (allowing your back to arch). See if you can get a real sense of reaching down into the leg from the pelvis, through the hip joint, through the knee, and out through the centre of the heel. The power of the reach comes from the engagement of the pelvis. This is how martial artists power up their kick. They kick from their core. You will find this practice so useful for when we come to explore walking and going up and down stairs, especially if you have had hip or knee replacement surgery and haven't yet fully learnt how to trust and integrate your new joint.

Now would be the time, if you haven't already done so, to explore this exercise and progressions on the other side, being open to and respectful of any differences between the two sides.

Exercise 15: **Variations**

One of the reasons I love the stick work is that it is so easy to introduce an almost infinite number of variations into each of the exercises so that we are constantly 'stressing' all the connective tissue and joints. I use the word 'stress' here not in a negative way but in the positive sense of causing adaptions in multiple planes of motion so that we have a strong healthy spine and joints that can adapt to all the demands we place upon it to support our movement.

You can achieve this variety simply by exploring new places to put the bottom of the stick on the floor. Each position will change the angles and tensions going through the skeletal system and connective tissue. The possibilities are endless: position the stick a little bit more to one side, a little bit further away from you, or more off centre. These are just some of the variables that you could change in any of the exercises, but there are many others such as the number of repetitions, tempo, and rest periods.

Here are a few suggestions for the placement of the stick when exploring Exercise 15.

At the beginning of this exercise, I asked you to place the bottom of the stick somewhere around 2 o'clock on our imaginary clock. One way to explore variety for this exercise is to take the bottom of the stick further around the hours of the clock until the stick is pointing out to the side (3 o'clock) and then progressing to 4, or even 5 o'clock. There's no need to do lots of repetitions. Try a few movements in one position, and then change the placement of the stick by moving around the clock, but always give yourself time to sense the effects of each new placement in your hips and the different impact each angle has on the way your weight shifts.

I will show just a few of the possibilities in the images below (Images 80 to 84). The important thing is not to try and copy what I am doing but to explore the **easy** possibilities for yourself. It is a fundamental principle of this work that you should never move into pain.

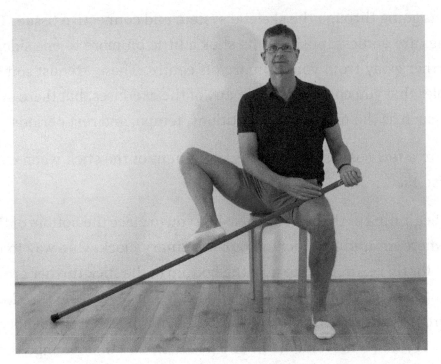

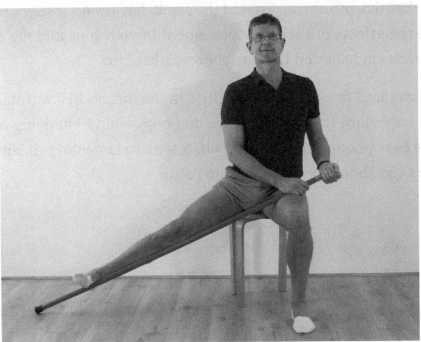

Images 80 and 81: Here I have positioned the stick to my immediate right or 3 o'clock. With this angle, as you can see, the weight shift is different, with less of a spiral effect.

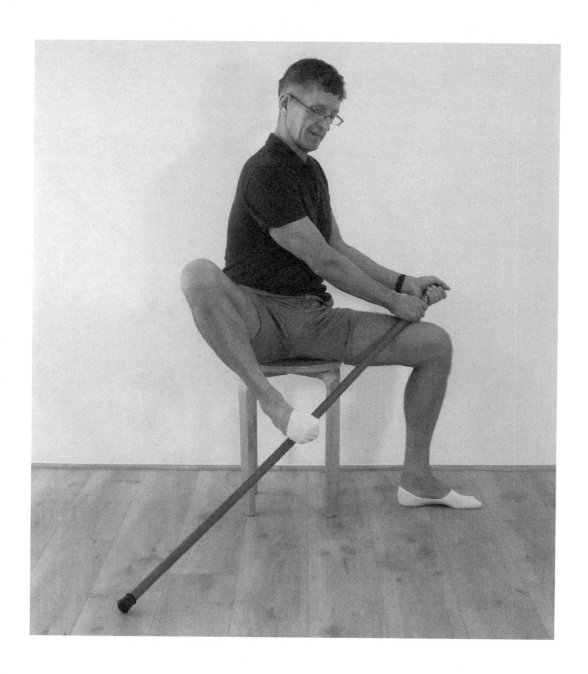

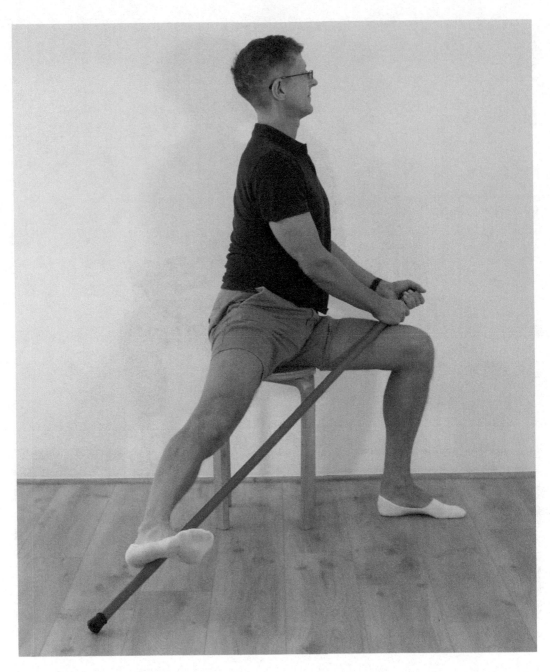

Images 82 and 83: Here the stick is angled more behind me towards 4 o'clock (seen from the side). When I explore these angles, I can definitely feel muscles fibres that I haven't used in a while being challenged.

Summary

This chapter has focused on developing the mobility and strength of your hips, knees, and feet and integrating their use into the movement of the spine and pelvis while seated.

Later, I will show you how you can use what you have learnt here to improve your walking and balance.

However, before you proceed to the next chapter, which is all about the spine, you might wish to pause for a moment and take a few steps around your room and notice how your newly invigorated legs feel and sense the weight transfer from one leg to the other.

5 / CIRCLES

Circles with the stick are one of the easiest, most pleasurable, and yet most powerful ways of introducing healthy stress into your spine. They bring together side-bending, flexion, extension, and rotation in multiple planes of motion, and you can use them to integrate vision and weight-shifting around the sit bones. I love them. My students love them. They feel so nice to do and from any point of view they are a fabulous way of introducing a huge healthy dollop of movement into some movement-starved spines. Once you understand the basics of the exercise, the possible variations are endless.

Let's dive straight into a circle and you will quickly understand what I mean.

Exercise 16: Circles

Come to sit at the front of your chair, widen your feet and knees, and hold the stick in front of you with both hands level with the top of your breastbone. Place the bottom of the stick forward of your feet (Image 84).

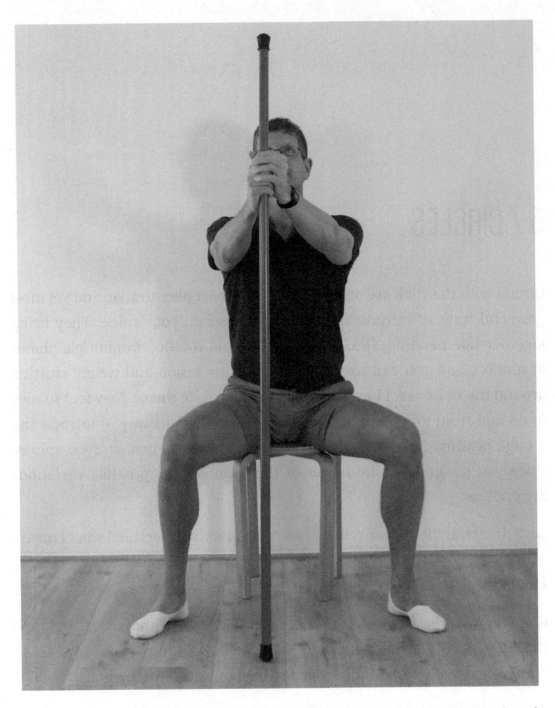

Image 84: One possible start position for circles. Here shown with two hands on the stick, but one-handed circles are a great variation too. Don't get hung up on trying to find 'the exact place' to put the bottom of the stick because, as explained in the text, there are multiple possibilities to explore.

Imagine you are stirring the most enormous pan of paella (or porridge for those who don't like paella!) and begin to trace a big circle with the stick.

As you reach out and away from you with the stick, look towards the top of the stick. As you circle back, bring your head and eyes down. Do several circles in one direction and then reverse the direction (Images 85 to 90).

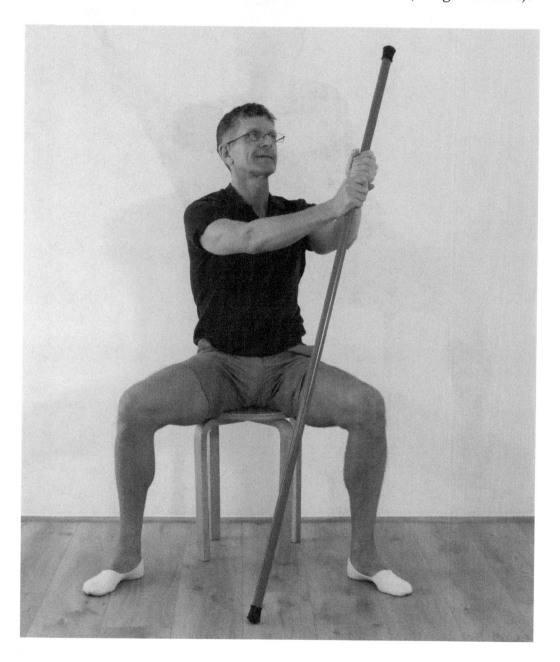

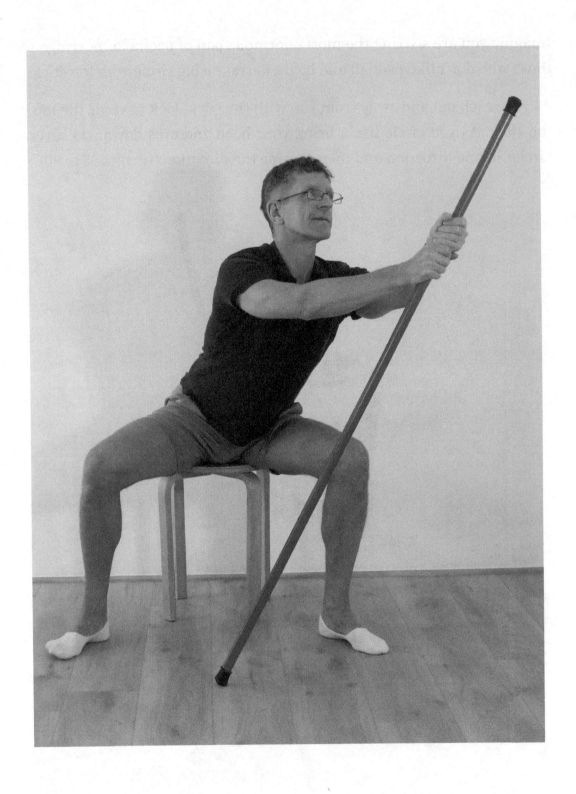

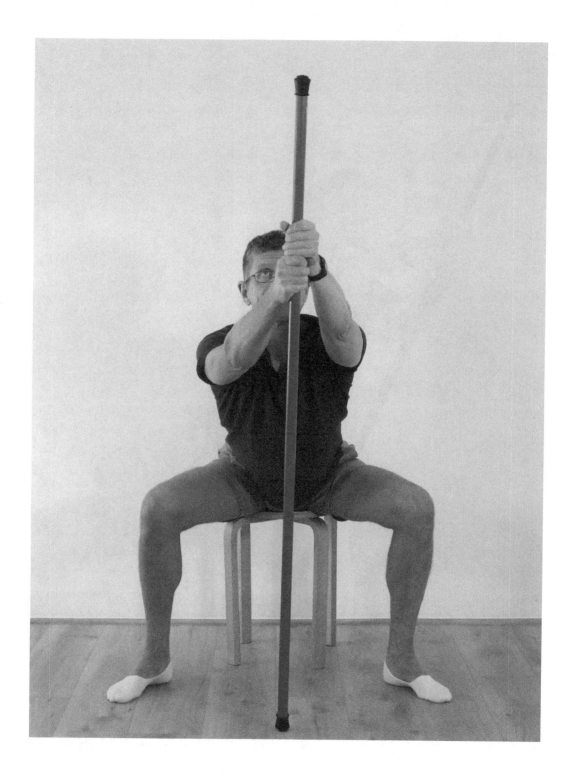

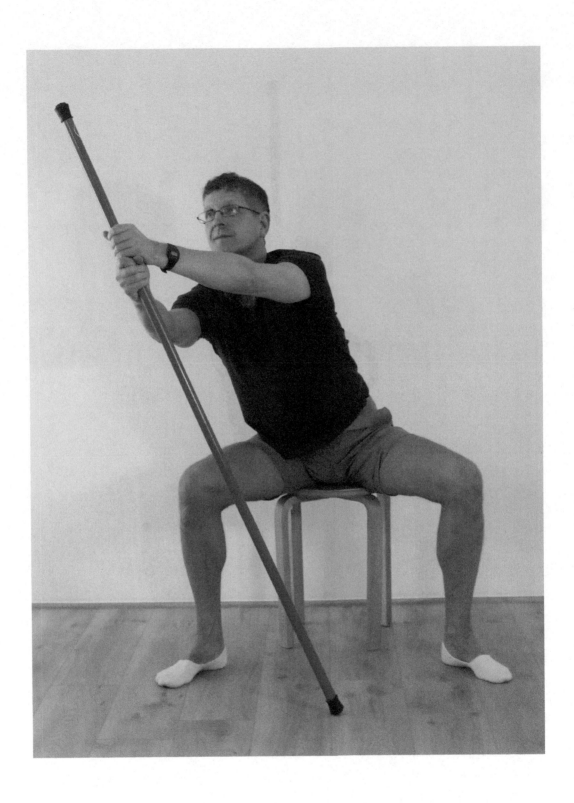

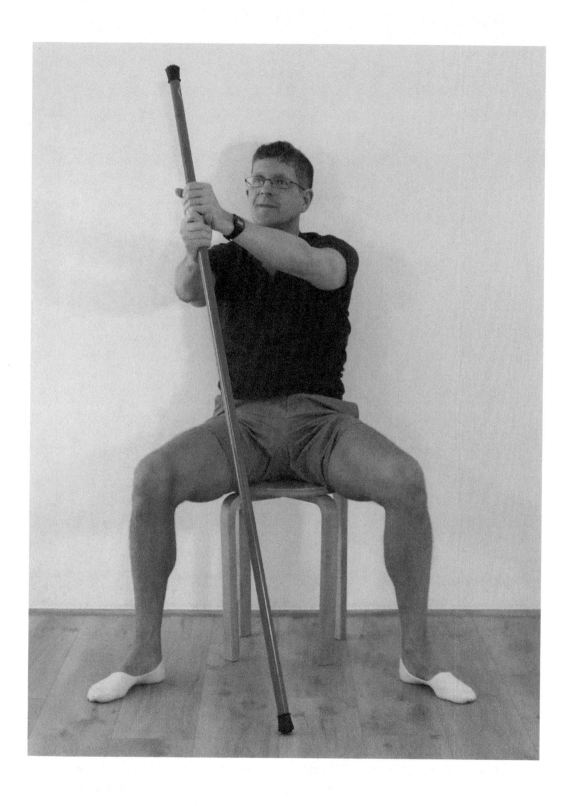

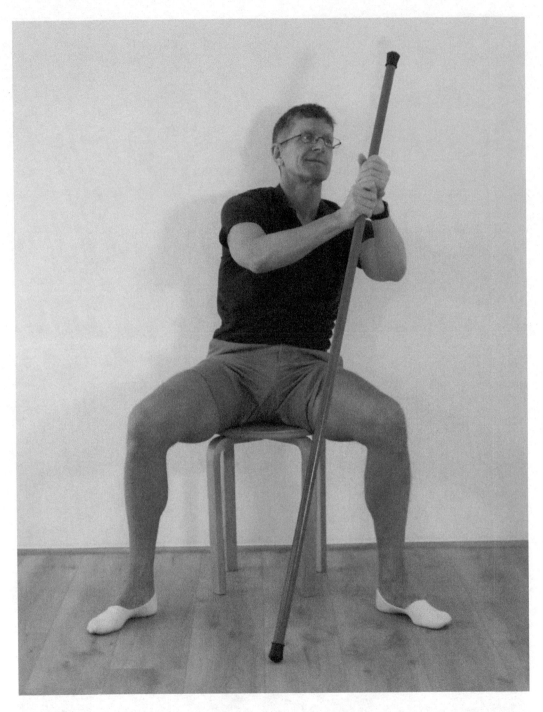

Images 85 to 90: A circle. One way of making these circles would be to keep the body completely still and just move the arms. However, we want to use your middle. Look at the way I am keeping my arms mostly passive, and the circle is coming from how I am using my pelvis and spine.

Sometimes, when I first teach this exercise to a student who hasn't been used to movement for some time, they try to make the circles by simply bending and straightening the arms and keeping their middle rock solid, which isn't the idea at all.

The arms are really just connecting you to the stick, and the idea of course is that the movement should come from your centre. So, allow your middle to move. If you can do this, you will feel some amazing changes taking place in the ribs, spine, and pelvis as your weight shifts around the seat of your chair (Images 91 to 95).

Another image I use with my students is the idea that they are sitting on a roller coaster and to enjoy the ride. Somehow this image gives them permission to let themselves move more and to abandon habits of self-restraint.

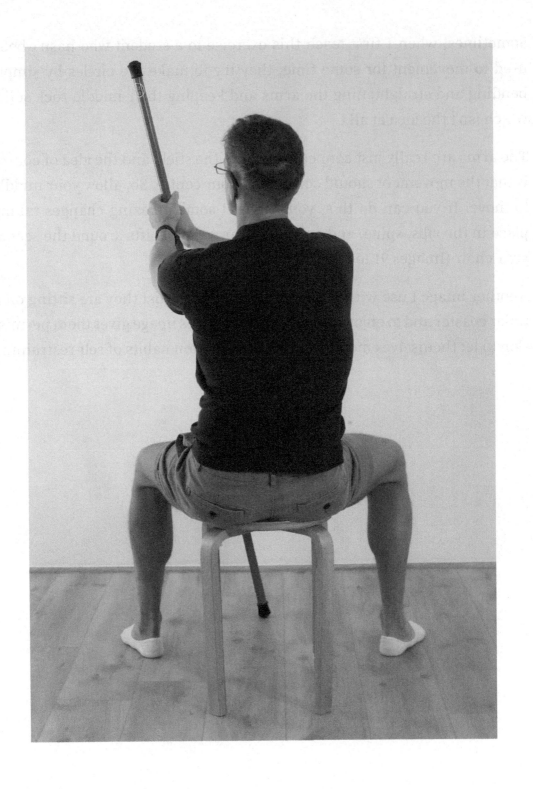

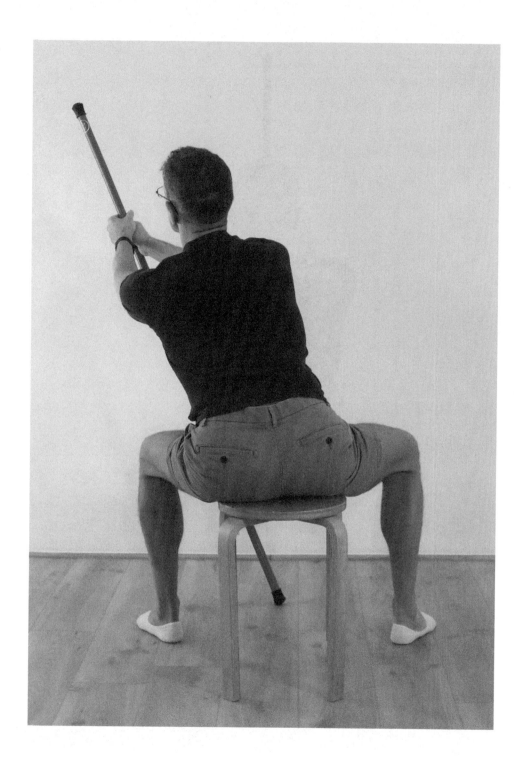

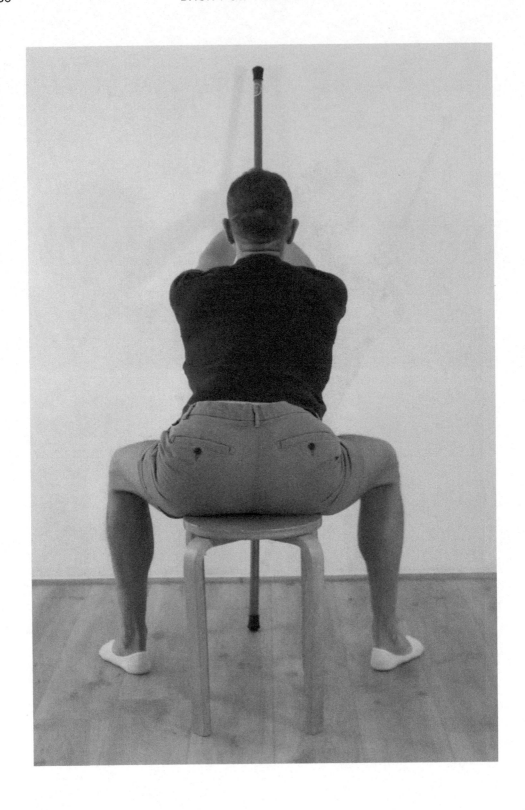

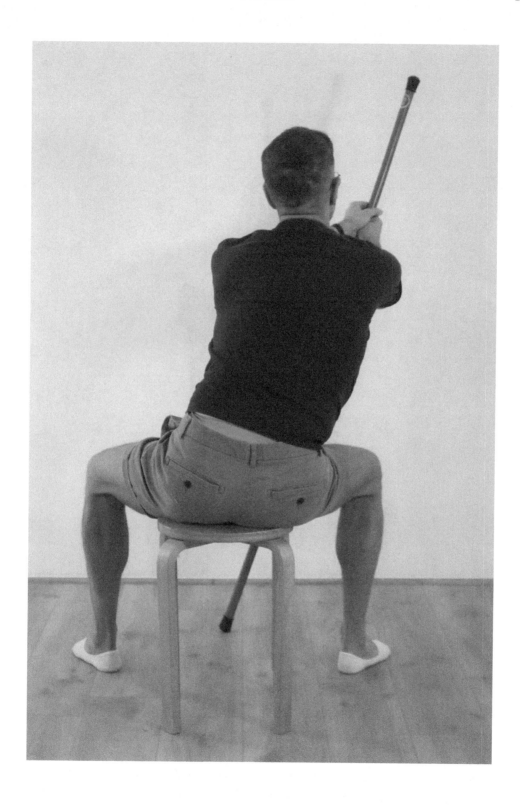

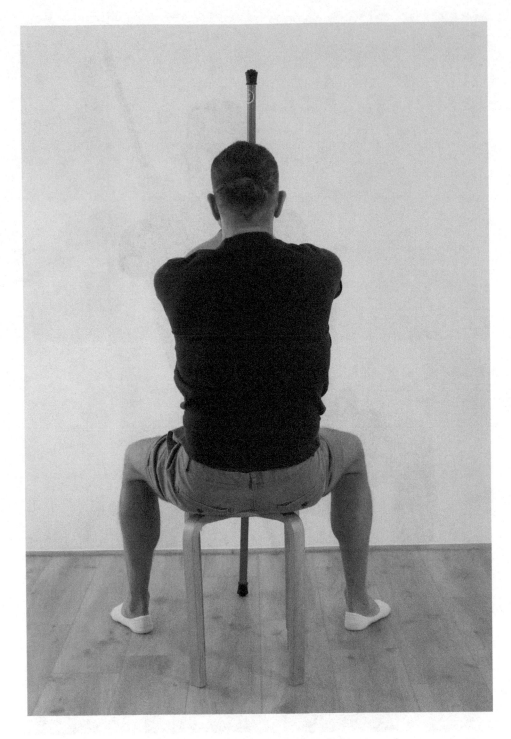

Images 91 to 95: Circles seen from behind. Notice the constant weight shift possible through the sit bones and the arching and curling of the spine. It's a movement that always feels delicious.

You will notice, too, that this exercise gives you the opportunity to practise your arching and curling but in more dynamic ways.

As you reach out in front of you with the stick, you are arching the spine. As you bring the stick towards you, you are curling the spine. With time and practice you will soon be fully initiating the circles from your pelvic power-house. The initial temptation will be to move the stick from your hands and your grip will be quite firm, but as you shift the intention to moving from your centre, you will be able to keep your hands super soft.

Exercise 16: Variations

Because the possibilities are endless, when I teach these circles in class, we only ever do three or four repetitions in each direction (clockwise and counterclockwise) with the stick in one position before moving it to a new spot, and I would encourage you to do the same.

For example, simply change where you have placed the bottom of the stick. You could, for instance, take if off centre to the right or left.

Or you could place it further away from you by a few inches. This will help you to lengthen the front of the body as you reach out.

You could hold the stick in one hand (Image 96).

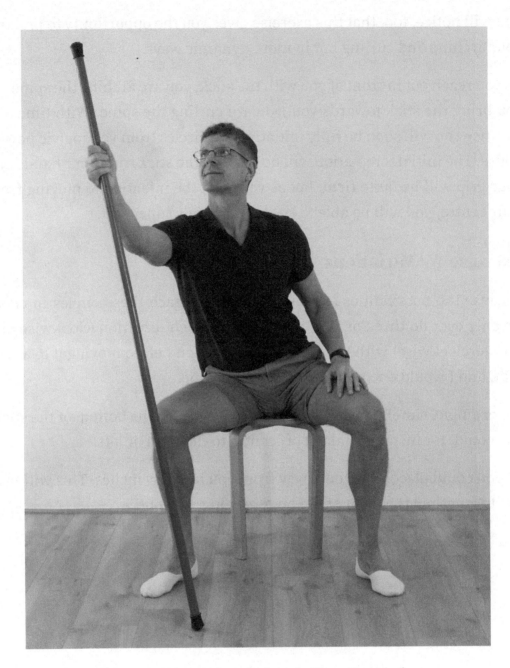

Image 96: A one-handed and off-centre circle.

You could vary the tempo of the circles, slower or quicker.

You can work with vision by keeping the eyes focused on one spot in the room while doing the circles or keep the eyes tracking the top of the stick. You could have one or both eyes closed.

You could change your grip on the stick. For example, if you habitually position your right hand above the left when you have both hands on the stick, change so that the left is above the right.

If you are doing one-arm circles, you could use a thumbs-down grip (Image 97). This will favour the extensors of the arms rather than the flexors.

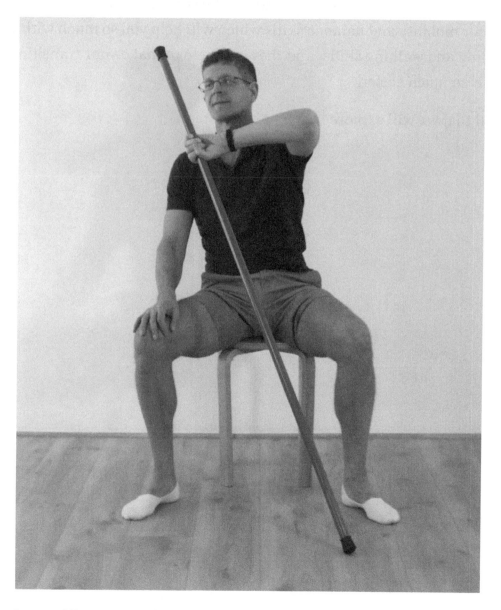

Image 97: An example of a one-arm, thumbs-down, off-centre circle.

Summary

Circles have so much potential to change your spine and get it moving.

Enjoy them and become curious about the movement possibility each circle creates.

As your centre adapts to the demands of these circles, you will be improving your mobility and balance skills which will help you so much with your standing and walking skills, and they will help to make your transition off a chair so much easier.

A skill that we will explore in the next chapter.

6 / COMING TO STAND EFFORTLESSLY

When I teach this vital functional skill to my students in class, they are often amazed at the end of the lesson when I point out to them that they have just performed something like 10 to 15 squats.

I think that the feeling of pleasant surprise comes because it hasn't felt to them physically as if they have put all that effort in, and that really is the point.

Getting up and down from a chair should feel almost effortless because it is a skill that comes from the way that you organise your movement and shouldn't depend on muscle strength alone. It is a skill that you can practise every time you get up and down from a chair or bed. A skill, that, if practised, will help to strengthen your muscles, and look after important joints such as your knees.

You may know many Boomers in your life for whom getting out of a chair now requires arm strength and lots of effort. We want to use the brain and legs instead.

Let's break the skill down and approach it slowly and safely.

Exercise 17: Coming to stand. Step 1: Knowing where your weight is

The first step is to sit on your chair with your feet on the floor. Notice that when you are sitting on the chair your weight is on the seat of the chair. You know this is true and can confirm it by simply lifting one foot into the air (Image 98).

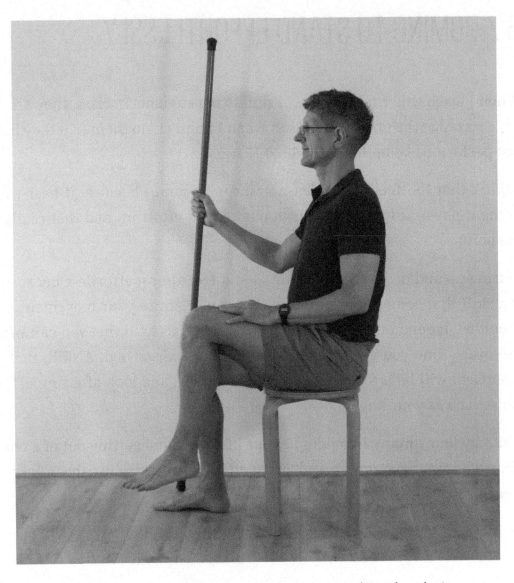

Image 98: I know that my weight is located on the chair because I can easily lift one foot from the floor.

It sounds so obvious, doesn't it? But you would be surprised by how many people try to get out of a chair when their weight is still over the chair and not over their feet. Consequently, they have to use their arms and a lot of effort to heave themselves up. We don't want that. We want to use the legs to bear your weight, so the next thing to learn is how to shift your weight from the seat of the chair into the feet in an organised way.

Exercise 17: Step 2: Shifting weight from the seat into the feet

Sit at the front of your chair and hold the stick with both hands level with the chest.

Check that your feet are light by lifting one, then the other, and then keep them on the floor positioned ready for you to come to stand.

Begin by arching your spine and look at the top of the stick. If you can't easily manage to see the top of the stick, then at least look at the spot above your hands on the stick. Keep the arms long at all times but not locked. The hands should be soft.

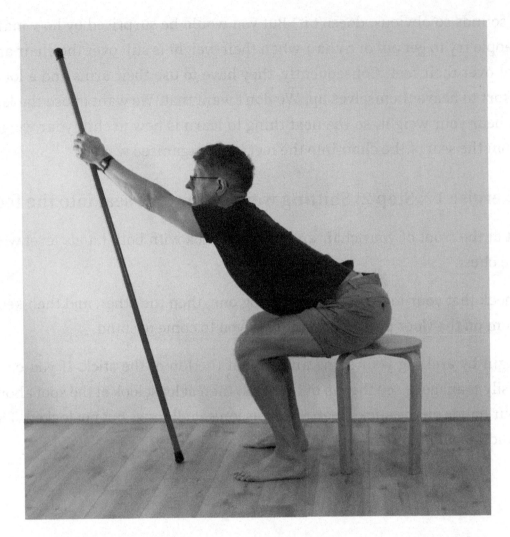

Image 99: Transferring the weight into the feet. Arch and reach the stick forward. Look up and keep your arms long but soft. If you look at the image closely you will see that my head has 'followed' the top of the stick forward. My head has come in front of my knees. I couldn't lift my feet now even if I wanted to because my weight is now in the feet and not in the seat of the chair.

Reach the stick forward and keep looking up at the stick (or your hands) and then return (Image 99). Do this several times.

As you become more confident and continue to reach the stick forward, there will come a moment when you have reached far enough forward that you will feel that there is no weight at all in your bottom and your weight has come into your feet. You will know this is true because if you tried to lift your feet now, you couldn't. Why? Because your weight has shifted from the chair into your feet. For this important weight shift to have happened, we need your head to have moved in space far enough forward and up so that it comes in front of your knees and not behind them.

As you reach away with the stick, always have the idea that you are going forward with the stick and your arms. You are **never** pulling the stick towards you. As soon as you let this forwards intention go and begin to pull the stick towards you, you will begin to fall backwards. So, breathe, keep your jaw relaxed and think: **forwards**.

In this step you are simply exploring your ability to transfer your weight forwards into your feet and back again. Please don't worry about coming to stand yet. That will come soon enough. Practise this simple exercise until you are very clear about recognising the difference between when the weight is in the seat of the chair and when the moment has come when you have transferred it into your feet.

Exercise 17: Step 3: Organising the feet and knees and activating the 'rebound effect'

Getting up and down from a chair should never be a fall, but it becomes a fall when a person isn't using their feet and legs in a way that supports them.

One way it often becomes a fall is when a person tries to get up from a chair and in doing so, they bring their knees together. It's an attempt on the part of the person to bring stability to the function, but it's a strategy that can cause havoc with the knees over time. It looks something like this (Image 100).

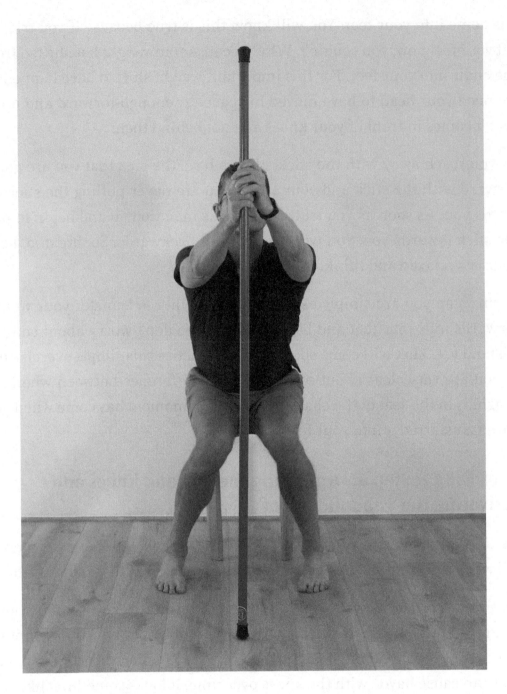

Image 100: A person will often try to stand by pulling the knees together. You can see that this puts a big twist onto my knees and if I tried to stand up like this it would put a huge amount of pressure into the inside of my knees. I would in effect be falling, and all my weight would be hammering into a part of the knee that is already vulnerable because of the twist in the joint.

When the knees are pulled together like this, and the person tries to stand, all their weight is falling to the inside of the knee as opposed to it passing through the centre of the knee. The risk of long-term injury to the knee is also increased by the fact that in this position the knee is twisted, making it very vulnerable to that sudden downward falling pressure.

To prevent this happening, we need to organise the legs so that they are optimally placed to bear your weight. Here's how to do this.

Before you begin to reach the stick forward, press your feet down into the floor and imagine that you are trying to pick up the floor with your feet. This will help to activate the arches of your feet and you will notice how, as you push into the feet, it causes a small movement of the knees towards your hip joint. It's a felt sense as you push into the feet that the movement **'rebounds'** from the feet into the knees and then into the hips. This 're-bound effect' helps to connect the ball of your femur, your big thigh bone, into the hip socket (see Images 101 and 102).

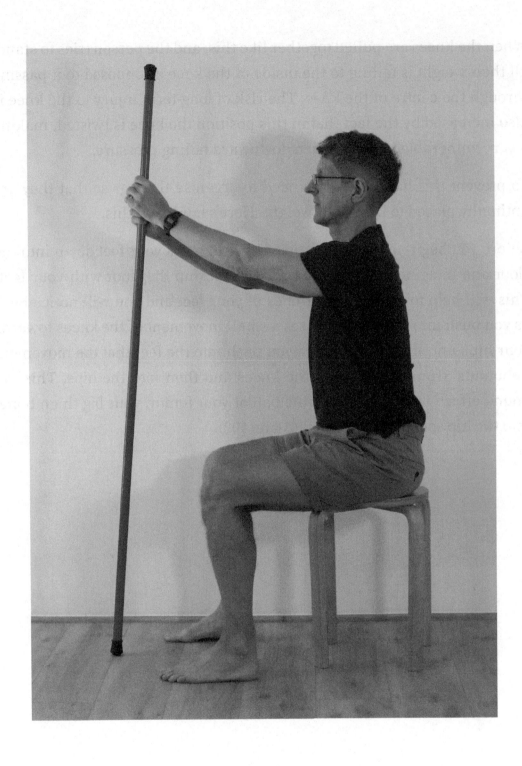

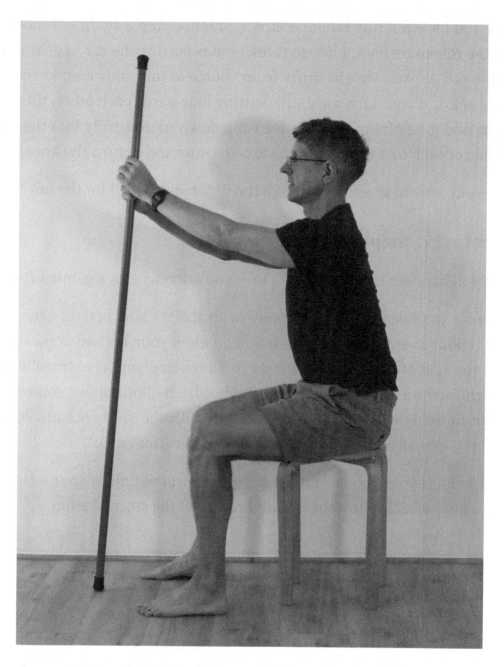

Images 101 and 102: The 'rebound' effect. If you compare the two images closely you will notice a small but very significant difference. In the first of the two images, I am not 'doing' anything with the feet. They are just resting on the floor. In the second image I am actively pressing the feet into the floor, and you can see how this activation causes the knee to move back towards the hip joint and pushes the bottom of the sit bones back. I am now ready to transfer my weight into my legs.

Once you have felt this rebound effect, practise Step 2 again but incorporate the rebound effect. I like to think of it as putting the car in gear ready for the off. As your weight shifts from your seat into your feet, keep your knees apart. If your knees are still drifting in towards each other, then you might find it helpful to think of pressing down more firmly into the little toe side of each foot to stop the ankle collapsing and in turn the knee.

Take your time to practise this step. It will serve you well for the next step.

Exercise 17: Step 4: Lift off!

Once you have put together Steps 1 to 3, you are ready for a gentle lift-off.

In Step 4 you keep reaching forward with the stick as before, activating your rebound, until you feel the moment when your bottom comes away from the seat of the chair. It will do this provided you have travelled far enough forward with the stick and the head. The bottom just follows. To return to the seat, keep reaching forward with the stick, but allow your bottom to return to find contact with your chair (Image 103).

Once you feel your pelvis contacting your chair, then allow your weight to fully transfer back onto your seat and return to the start position.

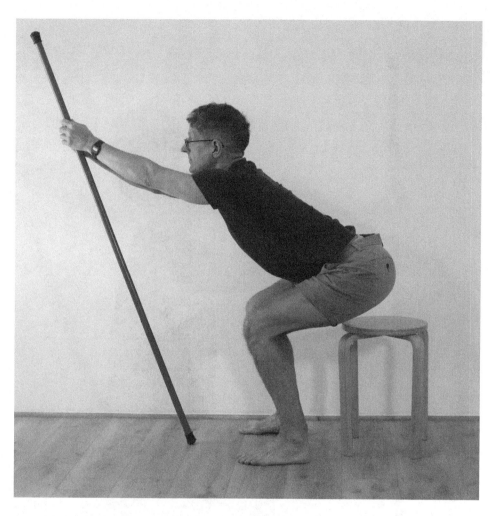

Image 103: Lift off! Notice how my head is forward of my knees. It's a sense always of the head going forward and up. The same is true of reversing the movement to sit back down. Don't think of going down but think of going forward, even as you are allowing your pelvis to reverse backwards.

Exercise 17: Step 5: Coming to stand

In this progression, you do everything as before but, once you feel that your bottom has come away from the seat, then just think of your bottom coming straight forward. And then *bingo,* you are standing! (Images 104 to 108)

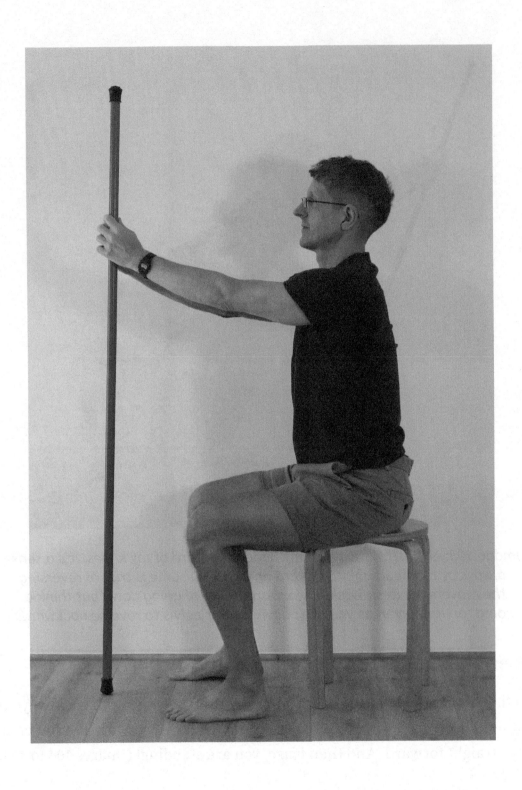

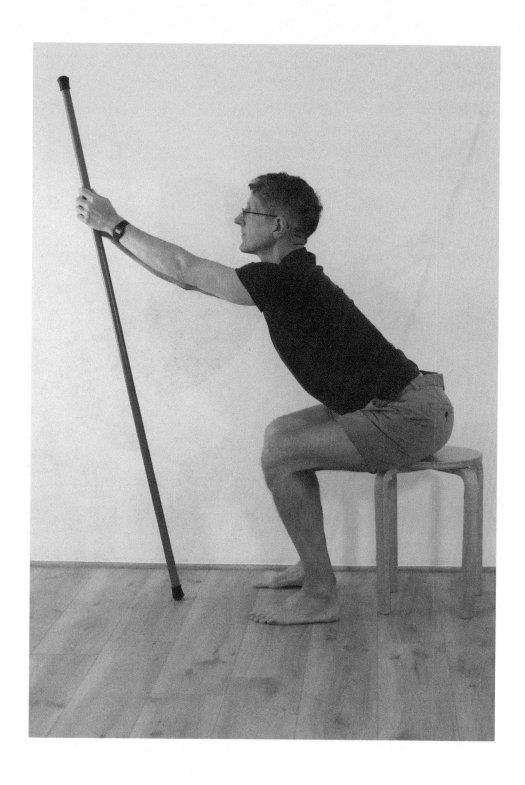

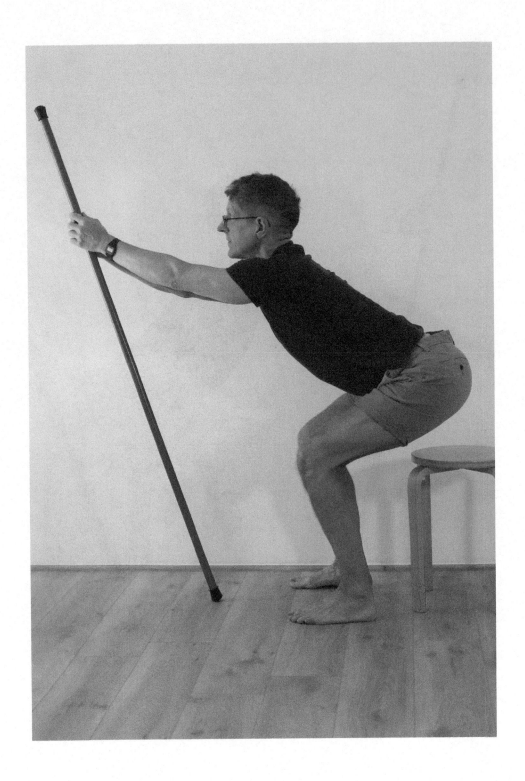

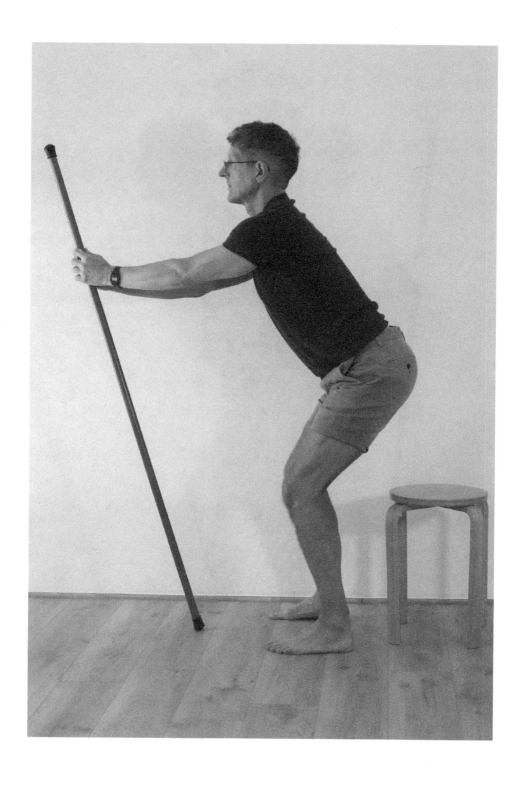

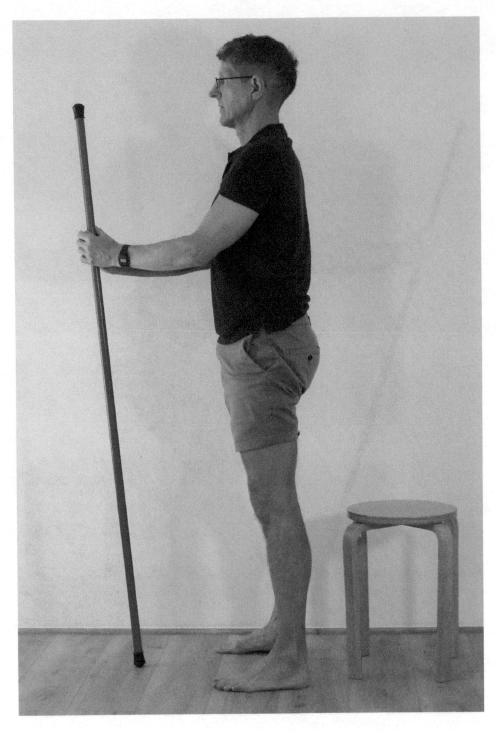

Images 104 to 108: The full sequence of coming to stand. At all times the head is going forward and up, and you are never pulling the stick towards you.

Take a moment to enjoy the view! Make sure you are standing upright. To sit back down again we reverse the steps.

Exercise 17: Step 6: Going forward to go down

Maybe this will sound odd when you first hear it, but it will make perfect sense when you have felt it. The trick to sitting down is to not think of going down but to think of going forward. It's exactly what you did to come up to stand but reversing the steps.

Once you have come to standing, begin to reach forward again with the stick and keep looking towards the top of the stick.

Keep the feet and legs active, and as you reach forward with the stick, allow your bottom to move backwards. There will come a moment as you reach forward that you can feel the bottom lightly contacting the seat of the chair. When it does you transfer your weight back onto it (Images 109 to 113).

Dah-dah and drum roll! You have done it.

The trick now is to practise both standing up and sitting down, checking that you can do both without holding your breath or tensing the jaw and hands.

One of the things that often happens in class is that a person feels the need to look down and back to make sure the chair is still there and hasn't moved. Unless there's a gremlin in the room, the chances are that the chair hasn't budged and the need to look is more of a habit that a person has gotten into. Provided your chair was on a firm surface it's most unlikely to have moved and what you need to work on is having the confidence to look forward as you sit down and to feel the point of contact of your bottom with the chair. That's all the information you need. If you are constantly looking down or back to check, the downward movement of the head and eyes will change the shape of your spine and will actually inhibit your ability to weight-transfer effortlessly. Keep looking forward and imagine rather that you have eyes in your sit bones.

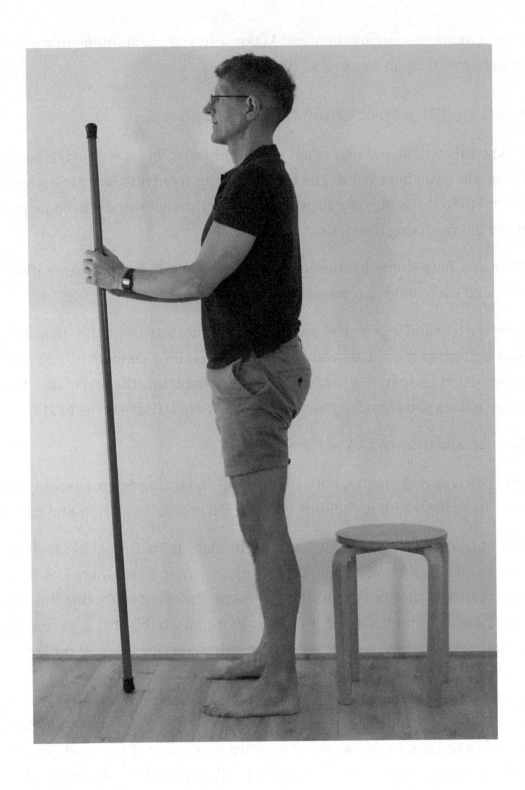

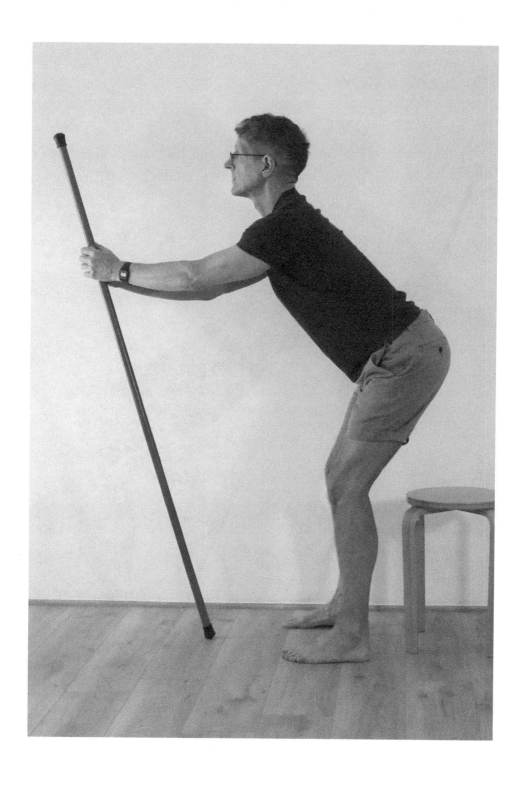

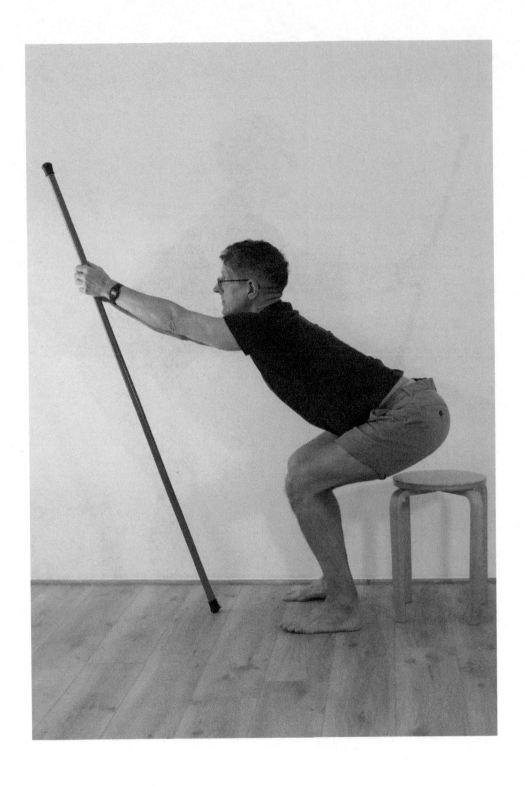

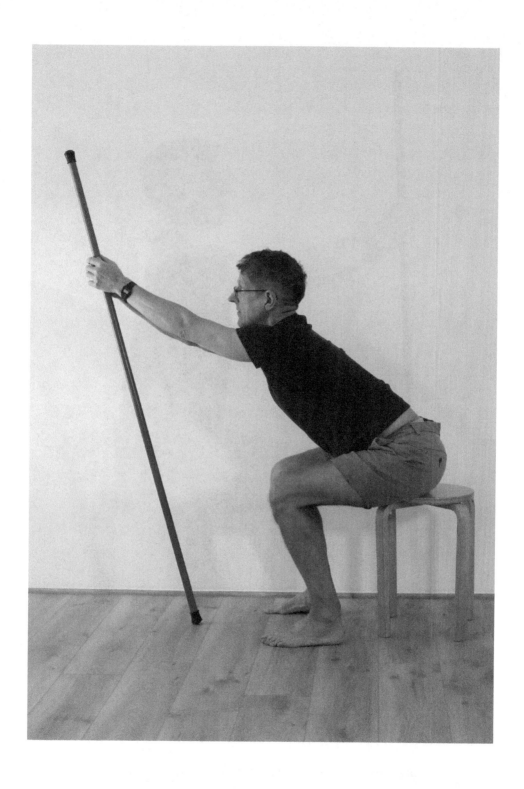

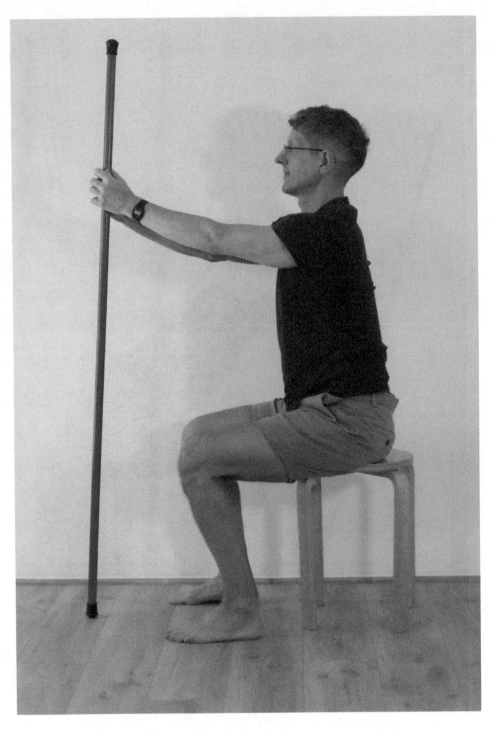

Images 109 to 113: To sit down reach forward.

Exercise 17: Step 7: Standing up and down with long arms

The use of the stick and the reaching of the arms is great for helping you to get the sense of the head constantly going forward as you make the transition from seated to standing and back again.

The stick adds a sense of stability and gives useful feedback to you that you can act on, but you won't have the stick with you all the time.

Once you have practised going up and down with the stick and you have felt and embodied the organisation that is necessary to transfer your weight effortlessly, then it's time to have a go without using the stick. We will do this first using the arms to reach, and then with the arms down.

While the memory of using the stick is strong, put it to one side for a moment but imagine it is still there. Reach your arms forward at shoulder height and keep reaching them forward as if you were still pushing the stick to come up, only this time your arms are apart. To return to sitting, reverse the sequence (Image 114).

It's remarkable how even the idea of having the stick there can help you to find the required organisation.

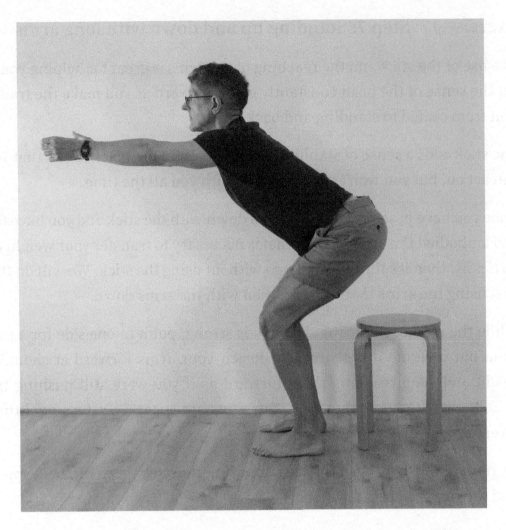

Image 114: Coming to stand and sit using arms to reach without the stick. If you imagine you are still reaching the stick forwards as you stand and sit, it will help you to find the organisation that underpins the effortless weight transference.

Practise this until you are confident that you can make the transition without holding your breath.

Exercise 17: Step 8: Coming to stand with the arms down

You are now ready for the final step which is coming to stand with the arms resting by your side. In this variation, you keep the arms hanging by the side. The trick, of course, as you learnt from using the stick, is to allow the head to go forward and up until you feel the weight come into the feet.

To sit back down, you simply reverse the steps. Think at all times of your head going forward and up, even to go down (Images 115 to 118).

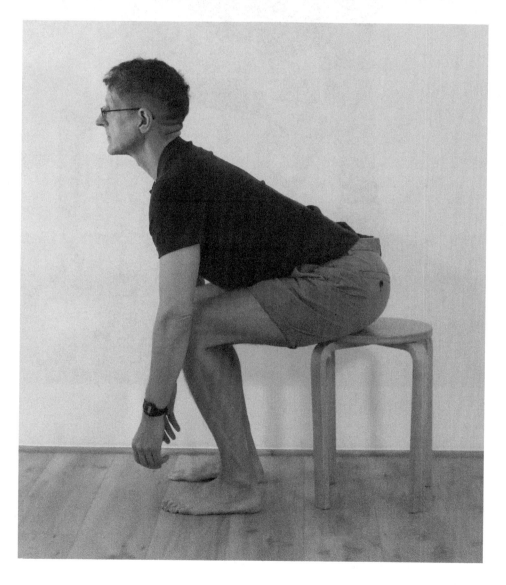

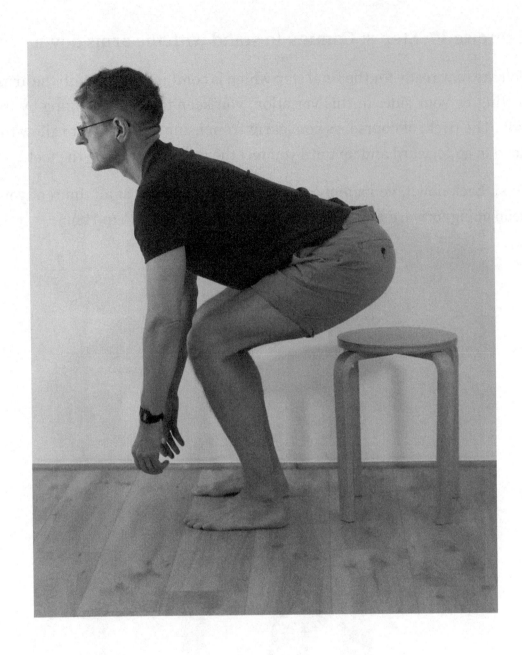

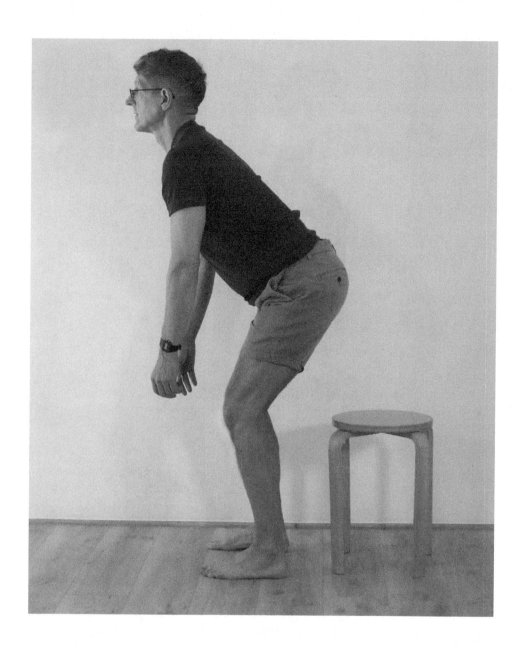

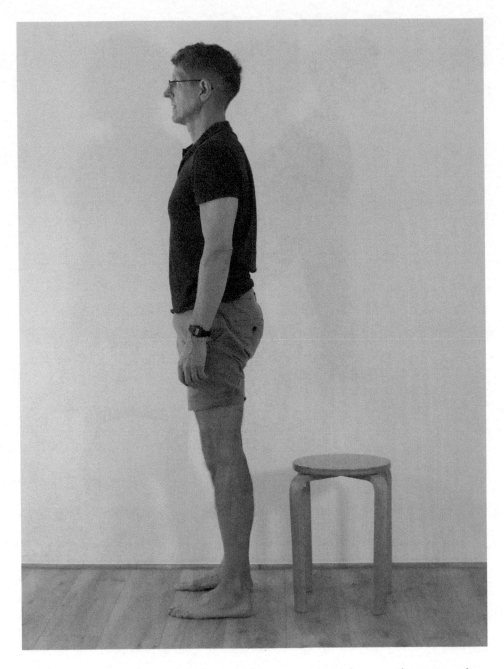

Images 115 to 118: Coming to stand sequence with arms hanging down.

By the time you have practised Exercise 17 and all its steps, you will have gained a deep appreciation of how it is possible to move through skilful weight transference. You will be able to reinforce this skill every time you use a chair.

Sometimes, however, it is not possible or practical to get up or sit down using both legs symmetrically. Sometimes we need to get up to one side using one leg more than the other to do so.

The asymmetrical use of our legs and hips embodied in this variation is a great way of exploring and identifying any differences in the way you may be habitually using one hip more than the other. Practice, with awareness, of the movements explored in the following variations will help to balance up these differences. This will be a great help for functional activities such as getting into and out of a car and when we come to look at walking and going up and down stairs with confidence.

Exercise 18: Landing towards one hip

Stand and hold the stick in your right hand.

Then begin to sit down, but this time aim your pelvis more towards the right hip joint, as if you wanted to sit down just on your right buttock but don't go all the way down (Images 119 and 120).

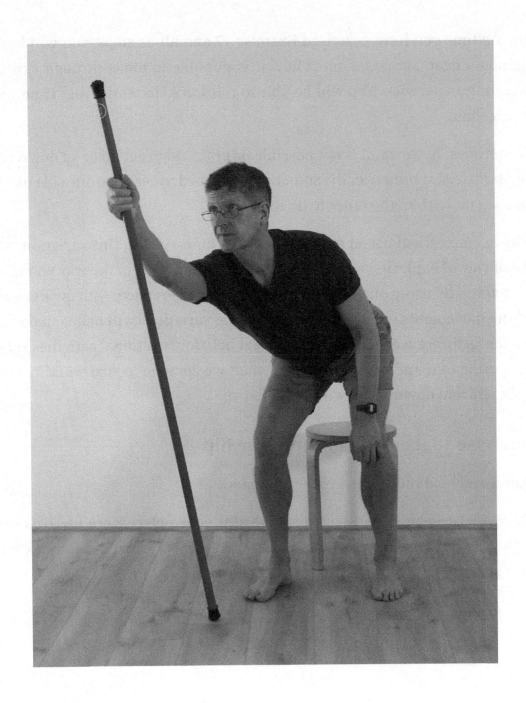

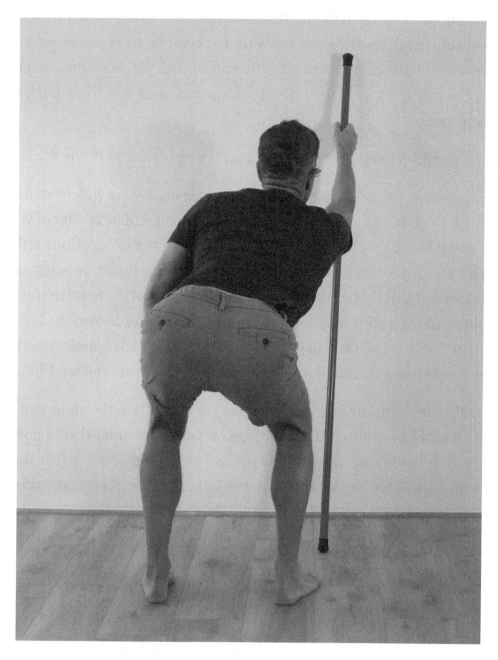

Images 119 and 120: Sitting down towards the right buttock. Front and rear view.

There's no need to actually sit. You are first exploring how far you can comfortably lengthen the right hip joint backwards, as if you wanted to sit down on that buttock but haven't fully committed yet. If you do reach the seat of the chair, it's only the lightest of touches, and you come back up to standing again.

All the time keep looking forward and up towards the top of the stick.

Ask yourself, as you are exploring this movement, is your weight really being borne by your right leg and hip joint? Or do you still have a lot of weight going down through your left leg? The answer to these questions will tell you a lot about your habits and whether you tend to favour one leg all the time. Obviously, in this exercise we would like the weight to be in the right hip joint and leg and it may take some time and careful work to build up your 'trust' in that leg and hip joint. You might find, for example, that there are moments when you suddenly 'veer' the weight off into the left hip or leg.

Repeat this exploration four or five times going down to the right and then explore a similar number of repetitions on the other side, sitting down to the left. In other words, moving the pelvis back and down towards the left hip as if you wanted to sit on your left buttock first rather than your two buttocks evenly.

What differences do you detect between the two sides?

Try alternating the two sides so that you sit back first to the right, then to the left.

After you have done that, come to stand and notice how the two sides feel.

Repeat this exploration with the stick in the left hand.

Then take a seat for the next variation.

Exercise 19: Coming to stand on the diagonal

In Chapter 2 you may remember that we explored how you can support the reach of the arms with the spine and the pelvis. This reach can also be incorporated into another functional movement such as coming to stand on the diagonal. Let's look at this now.

Sit at the front of your chair with the stick in your right hand. Place the bottom of the stick on the left diagonal (the second angle) somewhere in front of your left toes. You may well need to widen your feet and knees as you explore these variations to find where the foot and knee should be best placed to support you.

Reach the stick away from you on the diagonal, looking towards the top the stick. By now you should be very familiar with the idea of initiating this reach not so much with your arm but from the lifting of the right side of the pelvis. Push down into the left leg and foot to activate the leg and feel the 'rebound' effect. As you reach the stick, have the intention that if you were to continue to reach a bit further, this could and will bring you to standing (Images 121 to 124).

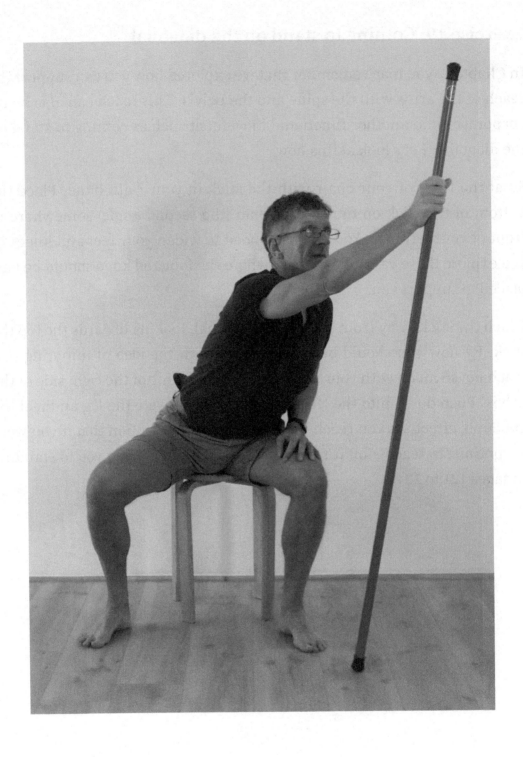

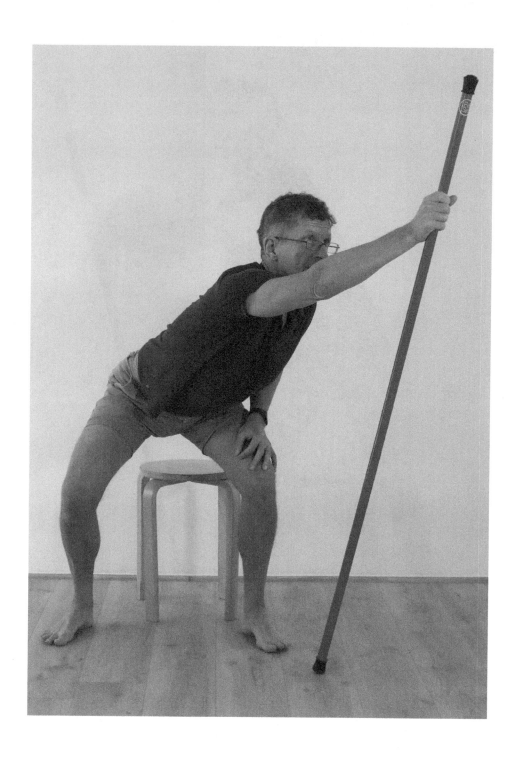

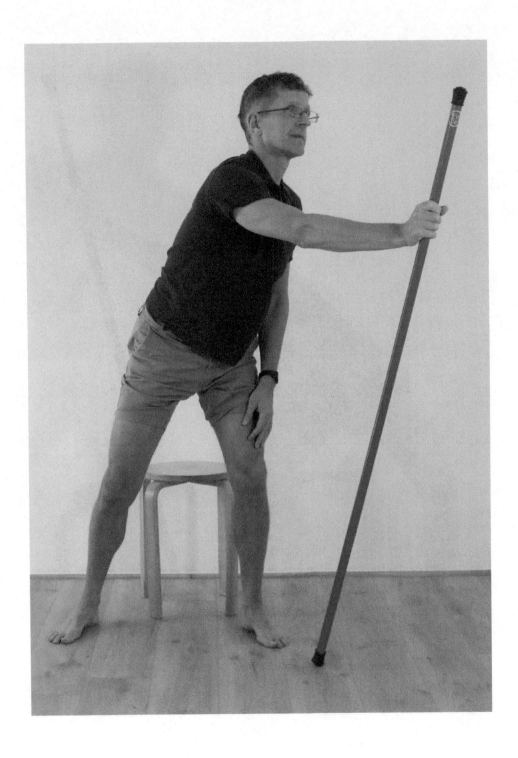

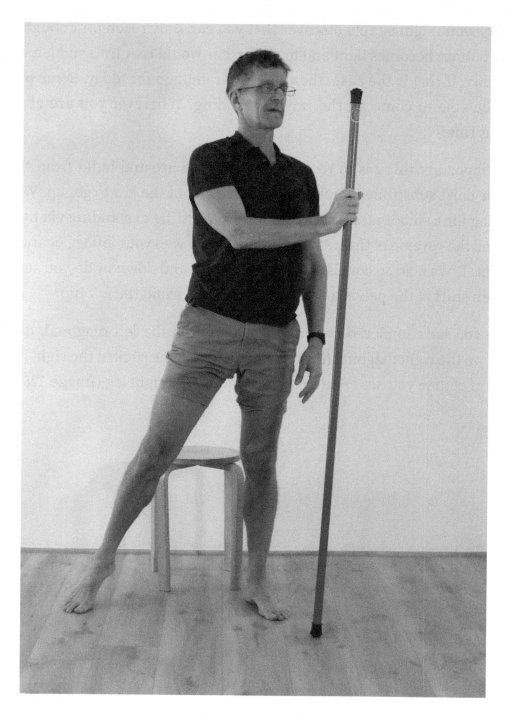

Images 121 to 124: Coming to stand sequence on the left diagonal (second angle) with the stick in my right hand. Notice how I keep my weight at all times on my left leg and hip joint.

At first you might simply discover that you can only reach far enough that your bottom becomes light and to go further would require a sudden surge of effort. If that is the case, then that is far enough for today. Some of you will be able to come all the way to standing. Wherever you are at right now is fine.

The important thing is to recognise where you are and build from there. Please don't substitute momentum or a tensing of the jaw to get up. We are looking for a smooth transfer of weight from sitting to standing via the left leg and the reverse of that. Pay attention to how well your left leg bears your weight. Does it do so consistently as you go up and down or do you sense a sudden shift of the pelvis to the right to try and avoid the left hip?

Once you have explored coming up to stand on the left diagonal, do the same on the right diagonal (first angle), still with the stick in the right hand. Here of course you are coming up to stand on the right leg (Image 125).

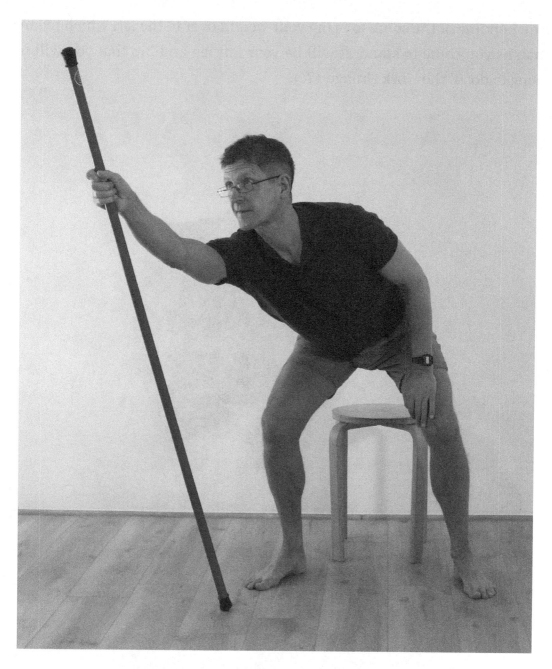

*Image 125: Coming to stand on the right diagonal
(first angle) with the stick in the right hand.*

The third variation would then be to have the stick, again still in the right hand, placed in your midline (the third angle). This is an interesting exercise to explore because, as we discovered in Chapter 2, there is a powerful side-bending of the spine to bring your weight over to the left which means that, as you come to stand, it will be your left leg and hip that you will be using to do all the work (Image 126).

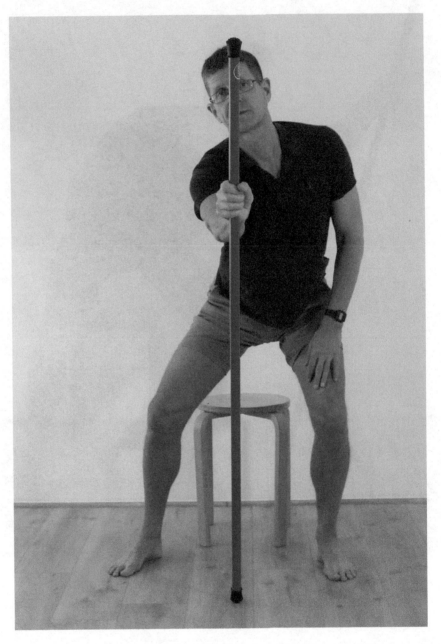

Image 126: Coming to stand keeping the arm reach along the midline. Here the curve of the spine to the left means that, with the stick in the right hand, it will be your left leg and hip joint that are doing all the work.

Finally, of course, these three diagonal variations can be explored with the stick in the left hand.

As you explore these, enjoy any discoveries you may make about any asymmetries you may have.

Summary

The material you have covered in Chapters 1 to 6 is the foundation of the Back for the Future programme. When I teach this material in class, I know that my students will have had within the hour a thoroughly good workout for their spines as one exercise flows into the other. More importantly, they will have begun to experience and embody the habit of initiating movement and expressing balance through their core. Because the material is infinitely variable, it never gets boring. There is always something new to learn or to practise.

My respectful advice to you would be to focus on and revisit the material in the first six chapters many times before proceeding on to the two focus chapters unless you are particularly keen to carry on. Spend a good month or so on it, practising the exercises at least two or three times a week. Your back will begin to feel so much more supple and available for movement, the learning will be immense, and it will stand you in good stead for the two focus chapters ahead.

In the first of these, if you are ready to proceed, we will look at standing and walking.

7 / STANDING AND WALKING FROM YOUR CENTRE

One of the issues that many people who have had hip or knee replacement surgery encounter is that, even though their surgery was successful, they are still struggling with their walking.

Often, this is because they haven't been taught how to integrate the new joint into their movement patterns and as a result they are left with the same penguin-like gait that they developed prior to the surgery. From the point of view of their gait, it's almost as if they haven't had the surgery at all.

This dysfunctional gait can put a lot of strain on the person's back and in turn, over time, can cause considerable pain and deterioration of the 'good' joints. The hope, that many of these people had, that the surgery would improve their quality of life and enable them to do the things they wanted to do, gives way to disappointment and a sense of frustration.

One of the reasons for this, I believe, is that the definition of a successful surgical outcome is rather limited from the perspective of movement. The focus of the pre- and post-surgery rehabilitation tends to be on the (very necessary) task of strengthening certain muscles groups and maintaining range of motion. The immediate priority after surgery is to get you upright and walking in the sense that you are moving forward on your two legs.

What's often missing are lessons that enable you to re-learn to walk in a way that integrates your marvellous new joint. and that will help to keep your other joints healthy too.

That's what we are going to explore in this chapter, which, of course, isn't just for those who have had replacement surgery but for anyone who would like to improve the way that they walk.

Most people, for understandable reasons, tend to think that we walk with our legs. However, if you would like to improve your walking it's important to walk from your centre.

On YouTube, there are some truly inspirational videos to be seen of individuals born with no limbs who can still walk, swim, and do so much more besides. They can do so because they transfer weight through their spines and pelvis.

By the time a toddler comes to stand and take their first tentative steps, much of the movement skills they need to transfer weight through their spines and pelvis to keep their head upright and balanced will have been learnt on the floor as part of their play and interaction with their environment.

In the previous chapters you have been bringing many of these movement skills back 'online'. As you practised skills such as side-bending, reaching, flexion and extension, your spines will have become more flexible. This improved flexibility enables you to express balance by initiating movement through your core in a way that adapts to your present needs. Let's look at how we can develop those skills in standing.

Exercise 20: Bringing the weight onto one leg: the 80 percent test

There are lots of ways you could balance on one leg.

For many people, however, it's a chaotic experience that they will often try and avoid. For example, they may lean against a wall or sit down on the bed to put on a pair of pants. There's no stability in standing on one leg. It's rather hit and miss.

We therefore need to practise the skill of finding balance through stability rather than chance, and that means organising balance through your pelvis and hip joints.

Stand with your feet hip distance apart, holding the stick lightly in one hand.

In standing you want to feel that about 80 percent of your weight is in your heels rather than the front of your feet.

One way of checking that this is so, is to ask yourself if you can easily lift the front of one foot keeping your heel down?

If you look at the image below, I can't easily lift the front of my feet because my pelvis is too far forward (Image 127). My weight is sinking into the front of the foot.

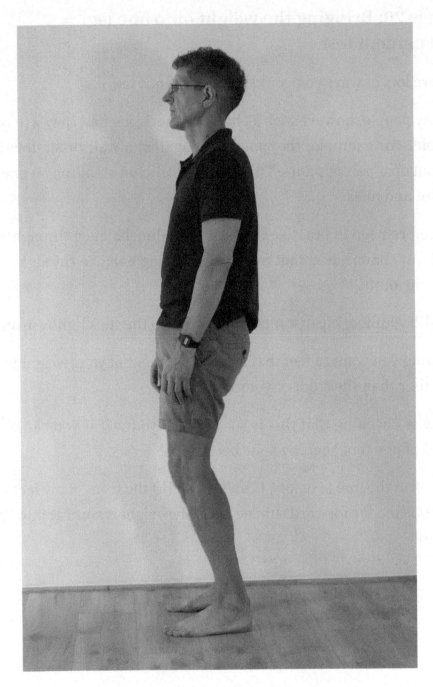

*Image 127: In this image I am standing in my 'sway back' posture again.
My pelvis is tucked under, my knees are slightly bent, and I am effectively
'falling', even though it may not look like a fall because I am still standing.
The direction is downwards. My weight is falling into the front of the
feet. I can't lift the front of my foot easily because my weight is on it.*

Equally, in the next image I can't easily lift the front of my foot because my head is too far forward.

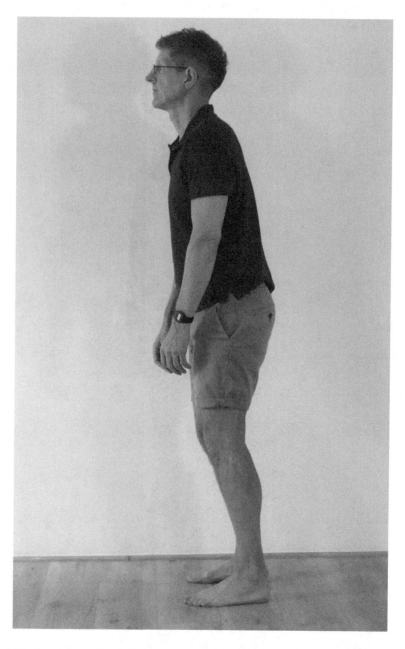

Image 128: Here my head is forward, and you can see that my weight is falling into the front of the feet. I am not supported by my pelvis and my lower back muscles are having to work very hard to stop me from face planting. It's not surprising that I am unable to easily lift the front of a foot.

By way of contrast, in the next image I **can** easily lift the front of my foot because my pelvis is underneath me and most of my weight, about 80 percent, is in my heels and passing through the centre of my knee (Image 129).

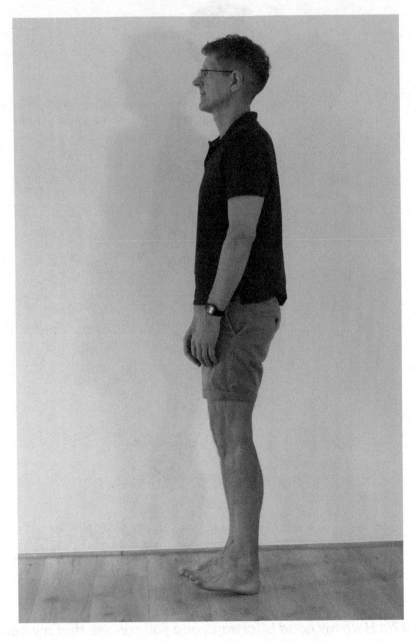

Image 129: Can you see that it is easy for me to lift the front of my left foot keeping the heel down in this image? This is because my pelvis is aligned underneath me, and my weight is going down through the pelvis, through the centre of my knees, mostly into the centre of my heels.

Once you have checked that your weight is mostly in your heels by checking if you can easily lift the front of one foot and then the other, we will begin by bringing your weight onto your right leg.

To transfer the weight onto your right leg, hold the stick lightly in one hand for balance, and initiate the transfer from your centre by having the intention that you are going to reach down from your pelvis into your hip joint, then into your knee and then into your heel and at the same time think that your head, the crown of your head, is floating up (Images 130 and 133).

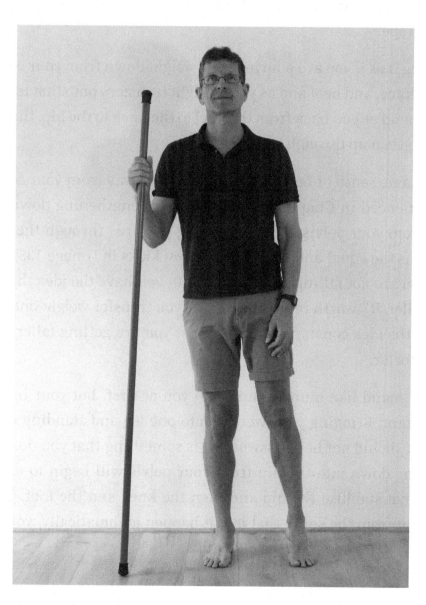

*Image 130: Transferring weight onto the right leg through side-bending.
Notice that there is no weight now in my left leg and my left heel is
lifted. This is because the left side of my pelvis has lifted as I reached
down into the right hip, knee, and heel. My left shoulder is lower than
my right and my head is able to stay floating on top of my spine. There
are two directions going on. A reaching down into the right leg and an
equal and opposite lengthening up through the crown of my head.*

What we are doing here is transferring the weight onto your right leg through side-bending. On the chair you practised this by thinking of squashing a grape underneath your sit bone. Here in standing, your leg is now the grape!

The feeling is as if you are pouring your weight down from your centre into your hip, knee, and heel and as your weight transfers onto that leg you will feel a rebound effect, back from the heel to the knee to the hip, that enables you to lengthen up through your spine.

It is that same sense of both ends lengthening away from your centre that you experienced in Chapter 4. Here, you are lengthening down into the ground from your pelvis and lengthening upwards through the crown of the head as the equal and opposite reaction kicks in (Image 133). In other words, you are not falling on to the leg, but you have the idea that you are getting taller. It's worth repeating this: as you transfer weight onto your leg you have the idea constantly in mind that you are getting taller or longer but not shorter.

This may sound like mumbo-jumbo to you at first, but your intention is all important. Bringing your weight onto one leg and standing on it is an activity. It should not be guesswork. It is something that you do. This idea of reaching down into the hip from your pelvis will begin to engage the muscles that stabilise the hip and then the knee and the foot, but if you approach it from the sense that it will happen automatically, you are condemning yourself to repeating old habits.

Practise this idea of reaching down into the leg and lengthening up through the spine and you will soon be transferring weight through your centre. At first you might just 'get it' for a nano-second, but you can easily build this up to intervals of five or ten breaths and then longer as your muscles and awareness kick in. Once you do get it, though, you will begin to feel very grounded and connected as you align yourself with the pull of gravity.

Trouble shooting

Here are two common errors to look out for but which are easily corrected if you practise in front of a mirror: trying to balance through the head and sinking into the hip.

Trying to balance through the head

People will often try and balance by tilting their head and shoulders to one side rather than side-bending through the pelvis (Image 131).

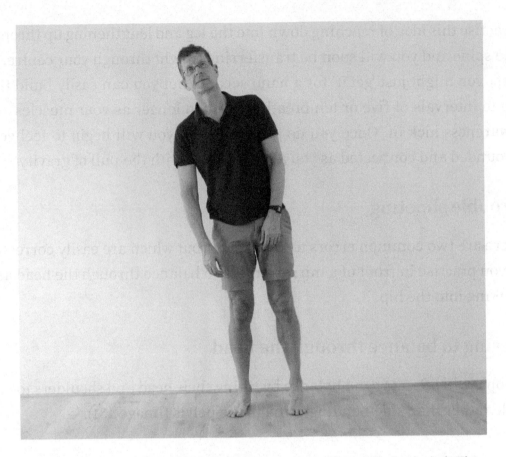

Image 131: Initiating the transfer of weight through the head. This is a strategy that many people use to shift their weight. My weight is certainly on my right leg as you can see from the lifted left heel, but the transfer has come from tilting rather than side-bending, and my head is now outside my base of support. I have become smaller, not taller. It is a chaotic way of transferring weight and is often accompanied by a tensing of the jaw and a holding of the breath.

As we discovered in Chapter 1, tilting as a strategy to transfer weight can increase your risk of falls and put very unwelcome strain on your joints. Your movement and balance should support your head so that you are free to scan your horizon. The best way to correct this is to use a mirror. It can be a little shocking to be confronted with the reality that you are not doing what you think you are doing, but the real-time feedback you will receive is invaluable. Practise initiating the transfer from the pelvis reaching down and allowing yourself to get taller as you do so. If you are tilting, you are getting shorter; if you are side-bending you have the sense of getting taller. That's the feeling that you are looking to cultivate (Image 133).

Sinking into the hip

Sinking into a hip as a way of trying to balance on one leg is very common. Instead of standing on the supporting hip joint a person sinks into it putting a lot of unwelcome pressure down into the knees (Image 132).

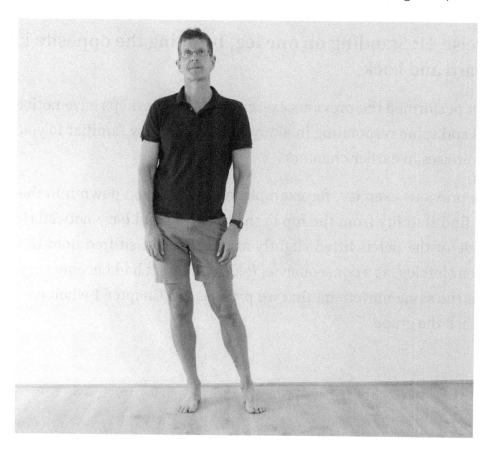

Image 132: Sinking into standing leg hip. Even though it appears as though I have shifted my weight onto my right leg and that I am able to lift my left heel, can you see that there is no stability here? I am very prone to a fall. My left hip is now lower than my right and once again I am falling. I am not getting taller as I transfer weight here; I am getting shorter. You can also appreciate from the image the sideways force this puts on the knee of the standing leg. Instead of coming on the leg through an active reach, I have simply displaced my pelvis sideways.

You can see from the image that when I sink into the hip, I am not getting taller as I come to stand on the one leg; I am getting shorter. If this is happening to you, the best way to correct this is to practise in front of a mirror, slow things down, and check your alignment. It will take time to build up the strength and awareness you need.

You should, of course, practise this exercise on your left leg before moving on to the next progression.

Exercise 21: Standing on one leg, bringing the opposite knee forward and back

As you performed the previous exercise you will perhaps have noticed the pelvis and spine responding in a way that will be very familiar to you from the exercises in earlier chapters.

In the previous exercise, for example, as you reached down into the right leg to find stability from the hip to the heel, you will have noticed that the left side of the pelvis lifted slightly as your weight shifted onto the right leg. Your left leg, as a consequence, felt as though it had become very light. This is the same movement that we practised in Chapter 1 when we learnt to squash the grape.

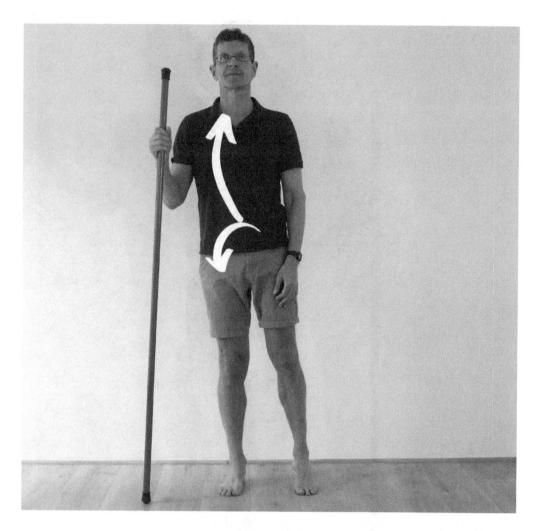

Image 133: To find stability on one leg there is an active reaching down into the leg from the centre. As your weight releases down into the leg there is an equal and opposite lengthening from your centre of gravity upwards. For me, it is a felt sense of pouring the weight from my pelvis into the heel.

In this exercise, we will practise maintaining your stability on your standing leg as you begin to move your other knee forward and back.

Begin by standing and transfer your weight as previously instructed onto your right leg. Maintain your weight on your right leg by actively **staying centred on the heel** and **slowly** move the left knee forwards and then bring it back to the starting position. As you do this, pay close attention to what happens to the left side of the pelvis (Images 134 to 138 side and rear views).

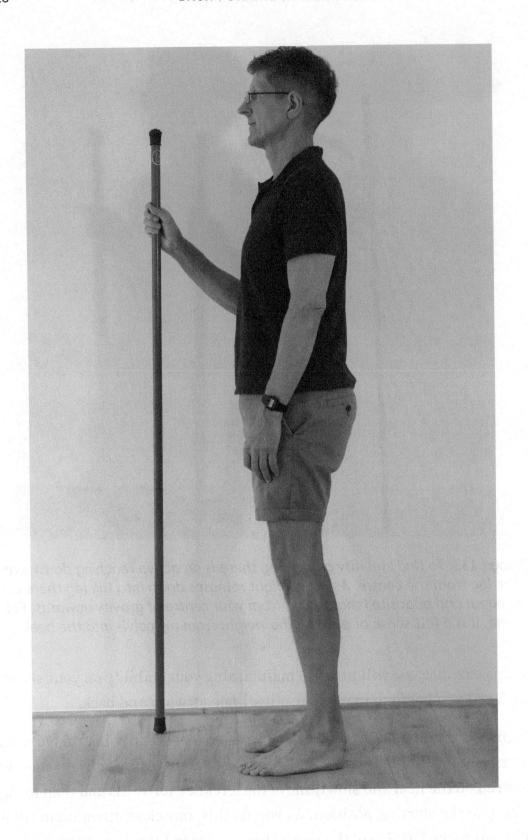

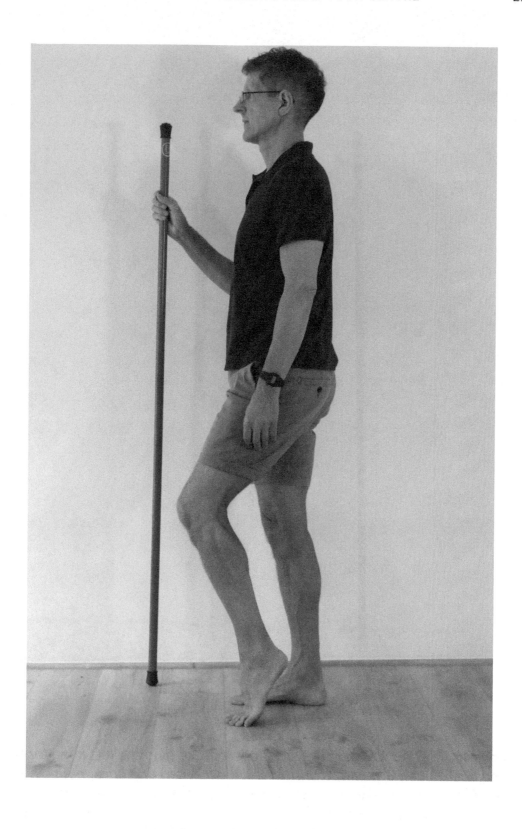

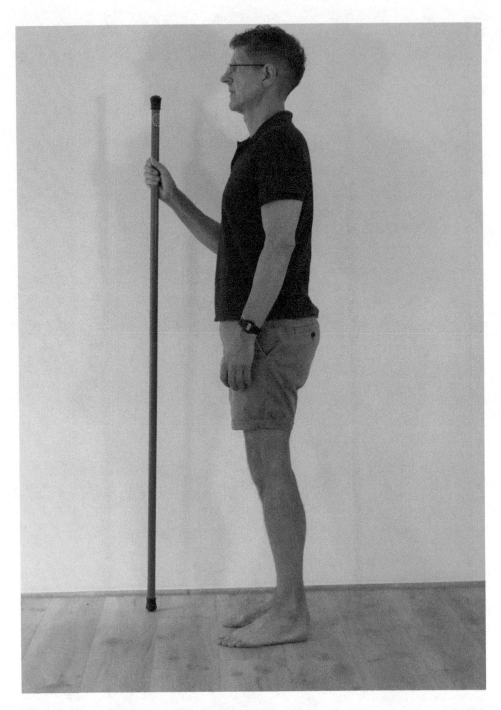

Images 134 to 136: Standing on your right leg, bringing the left knee forward and back. Side view. As you bring the knee forward and back, notice how the left side of the pelvis rotates forward and back. It is a small movement. Look at the button on the back of my shorts. In the middle image you can see how it has moved forward as the left side of the pelvis rotates.

Could you sense that the left side of the pelvis is not only lifted relative to the right side (because of side-bending) but that it also rotates forward as the left knee moves forward?

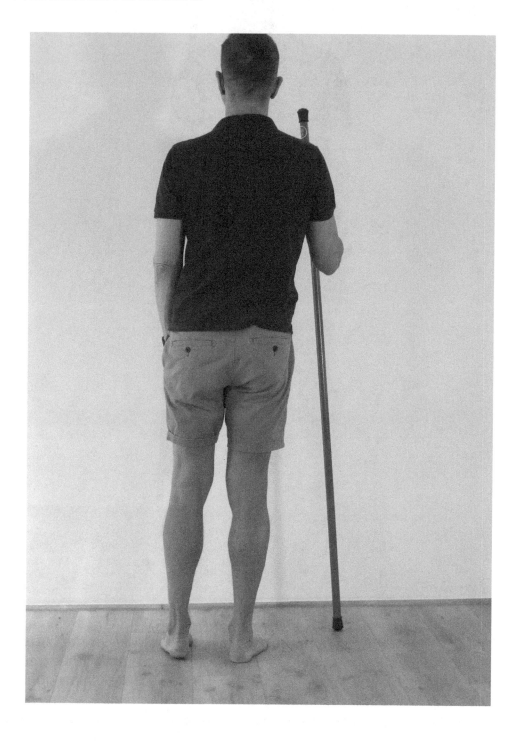

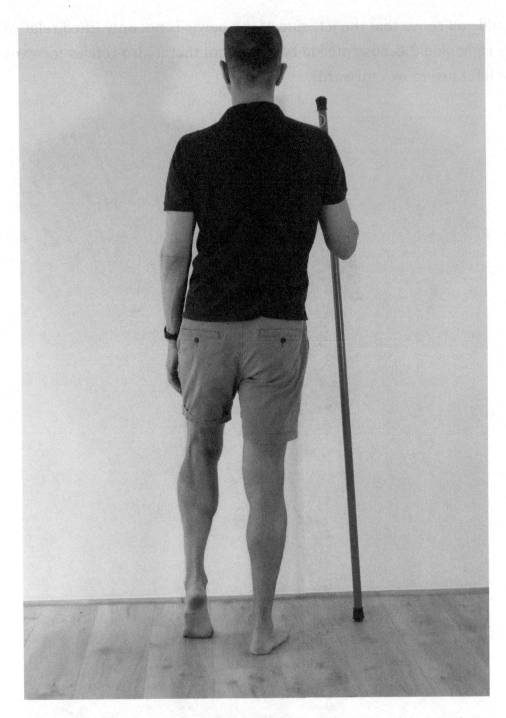

Images 137 and 138: Seen from the rear. If you look closely at the buttons on the back of my shorts you will see how the button on the left has rotated forwards. Notice also how in both images my weight is always on my right leg. The left shoulder is lower than the right. I am actively maintaining the reach down through the right leg and into the heel to keep myself stable on the leg.

This is a very similar movement to the one we explored in Chapter 1 Exercise 5 when we practised side-bending on the chair and differentiating the movement of the knee. You will remember that the movement of the knee forwards and backwards on the chair came from the pelvis and the spine. It may seem like a very small movement at first, but it is also a very important one. It combines your ability to side-bend and rotate your pelvis relative to your chest in a way that enables you to move forward in space while maintaining stable balance on one leg.

Once you have sensed this movement of the pelvis, the next progression would be to include it in your intention of moving the knee forward and back (the **core-to-distal** pattern). Now that you have realised that it is there as a possibility, you are going to use it quite deliberately and highlight it in your mind's eye.

Repeat the exercise once more, but this time you are initiating the movement of the knee forward and back from your centre.

Here's the sequence:

1. Stand on both feet equally.

2. Bring the weight onto the right leg.

3. Move the left knee forward, then back, allowing the left side of the pelvis to rotate forward and back.

4. Move the weight back onto both feet.

Practise this several times standing on the right leg and then explore the same on the left leg.

Exercise 22: Standing on leg and taking the first step forward

The next progression would be to allow the left knee to continue to move further forward to place the foot.

Begin by standing, holding the stick for balance, and transfer your weight onto your right leg. Once you feel stable and tall on your right leg, allow your left knee to move forward and to continue to move forward until the left heel peels away from the floor followed by the toes.

As the left knee moves forward, the left foot peels away from the floor and, once clear, will swing forward and place on the floor underneath the knee. This is exactly where we want it to be, ready to bear your weight as you transfer off the right leg. We will do that in the next exercise but for the moment, confine yourself to bringing the knee forward to place the foot and then bring it back, slowly, without actually shifting your weight onto the left leg (Images 139 to 141).

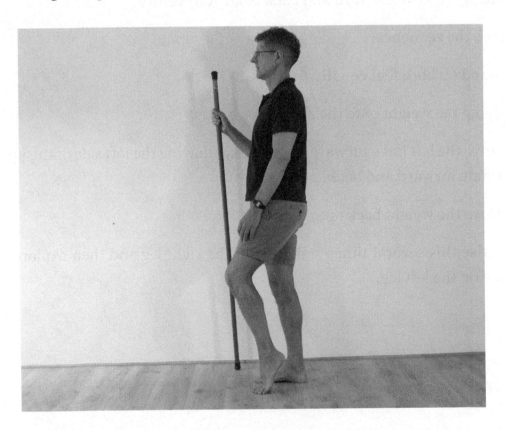

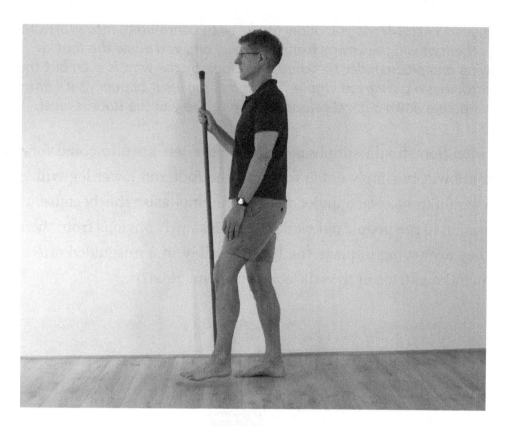

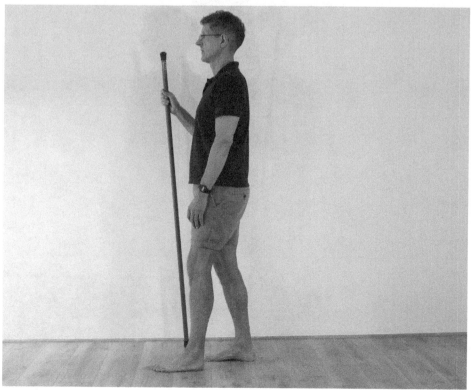

Images 139 to 141: As you allow the knee to continue to move forwards, the foot will peel away from the floor, and you allow the foot to swing and place under the knee. The floor, by the way, is even but the studio is a converted stable. The image makes it appear as if I am walking down a gentle slope, but I promise you the floor is level.

Your intention should simply be to allow the left knee to come forward. If you allow it to simply come forward, the foot and lower leg will swing like a pendulum to place under the knee. I emphasise this because it's not uncommon to see people out walking and it's fairly obvious from their gait that they are trying to place the heel, possibly in a misguided attempt to lengthen their stride or to walk 'correctly' (Image 142).

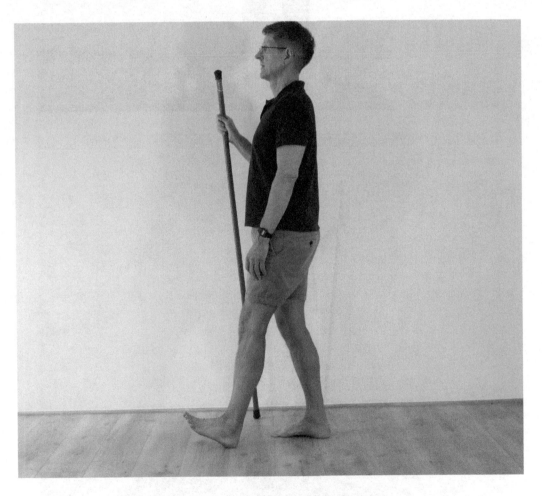

Image 142: An example of what trying to deliberately 'place' the heel looks like.

The sequence to practise therefore would be:

1. Stand on both feet equally.

2. Bring the weight onto the right leg.

3. Move the left knee forward, allowing the foot to swing and place underneath the knee. Then bring it back again.

4. Move the weight from the right leg back equally onto both feet.

Try this on the other side before moving on to the next exercise.

Exercise 23: Transferring weight onto the forward leg

During the course of building up this sequence you have been paying very close attention to knowing on which leg your weight is situated.

To begin with, this may seem a little artificial and like hard work, but this awareness is key to improving your ability to move well. As this skill of stable weight transference becomes more embodied, it will become second nature, a part of the way that you move. You won't always need to move as cautiously as we are doing in this practice, but there are times when the ability to move very deliberately and carefully are vital to your survival.

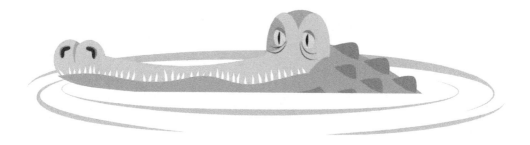

Figure L: Paying attention to your weight transference could save your life!

One image I sometimes ask my students to play with is the idea that they are trying to cross a river. There are some steppingstones that show a possible way to bridge the water, but some of these stones are not so stable. Take a wrong step and you plunge into the water. Even worse, one of these 'stones' may actually be a crocodile's head that you are about to step on. Danger, therefore, if you are not careful, lies ahead. The idea behind the imagery is that you should be able to test the way forward with the leading foot without committing your weight to it and be able to bring it back again without losing your balance. Students of tai chi or other martial arts will be very familiar with this idea of mindful movement. Toddlers too!

With this image in mind, once you have brought your left knee and foot forward as in the previous sequence, pause before committing weight to it. Can you feel the organisation required here in the pelvis to keep your weight centred on your right heel?

At this stage your weight is still on your right leg, hip and heel. The left side of the pelvis will have lifted slightly and rotated forward, but in terms of a side-view your pelvis will be positioned slightly behind the left leg (Images 143 and 144).

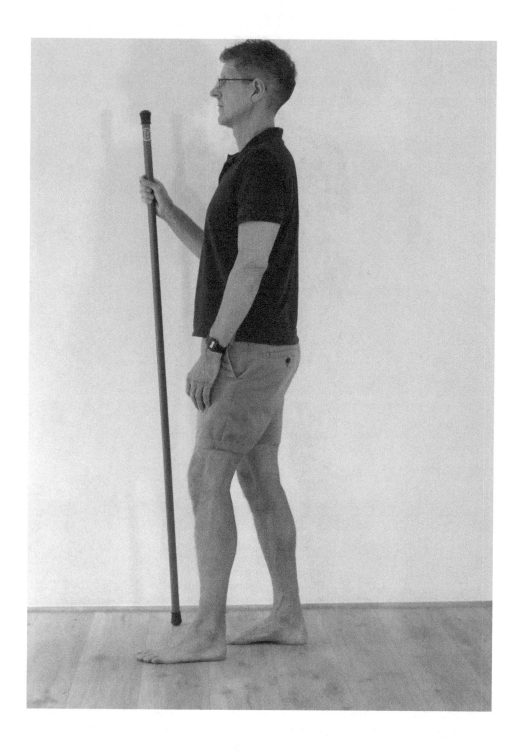

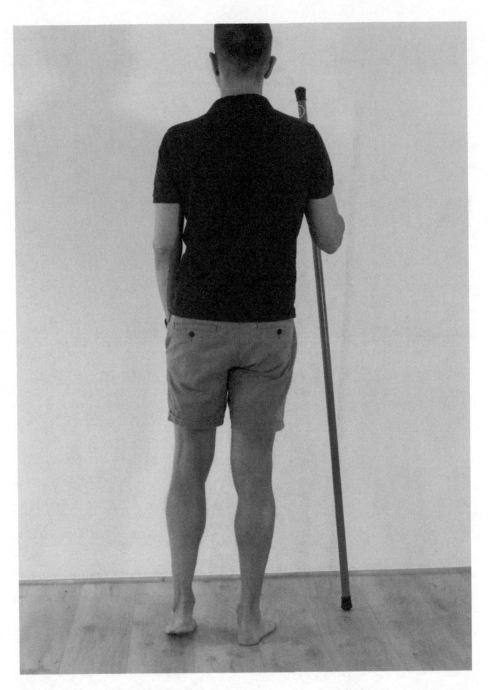

Images 143 and 144: Side and rear view of the moment before committing weight to the forward left leg. The view from behind clearly shows how my weight is on the right leg. From the side view, you can see how the left side of my pelvis is 'behind' the leg and foot. If you were to drop a plumb line down from my outer left hip, the plumb line would hit the floor behind my heel.

To transfer weight onto the left leg, two things happen simultaneously.

The first is the change in the pelvis. As you begin to move onto the left leg, you release the hold that keeps your weight on the right leg. That means that as you move onto the left leg you should allow the left side of the pelvis to release and now actively reach down to find the left hip joint, knee, and hip ('squashing the grape'). The felt sense is that you are pouring your weight from the right leg into the left (Image 133). As you do this, the right side of the pelvis will begin to lift.

The second element is the use of the right leg. As you release the weight off the right leg, press down and back with it. The muscles of the back of the right leg and hip will kick in and help to propel you forward and up onto the left leg. The right heel lifts, the weight travels along the outside part of the right foot and then travels over to the big toe just before the foot completely leaves the floor (Images 145 to 148).

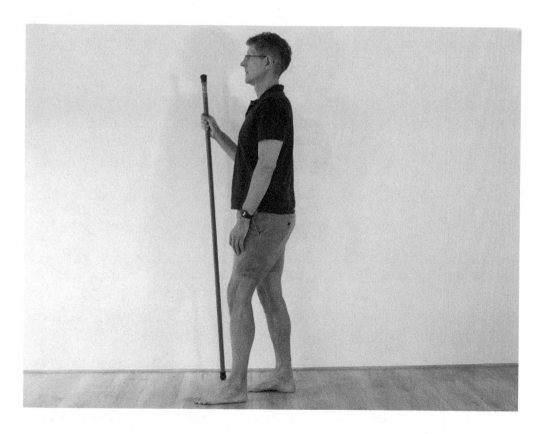

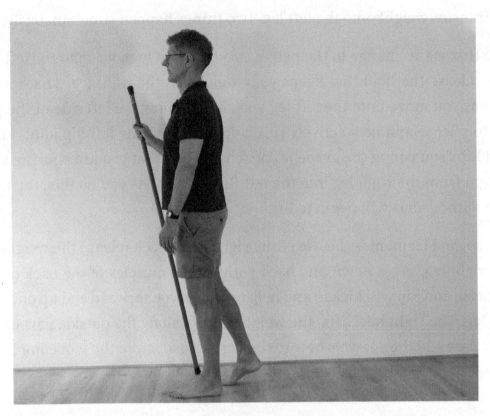

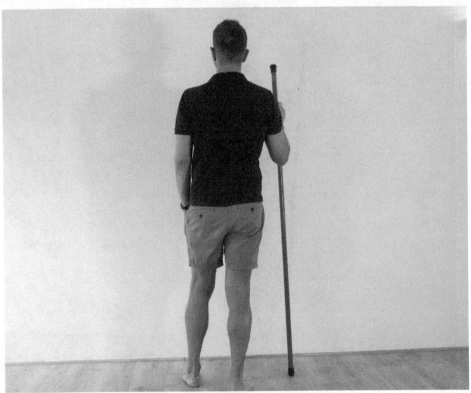

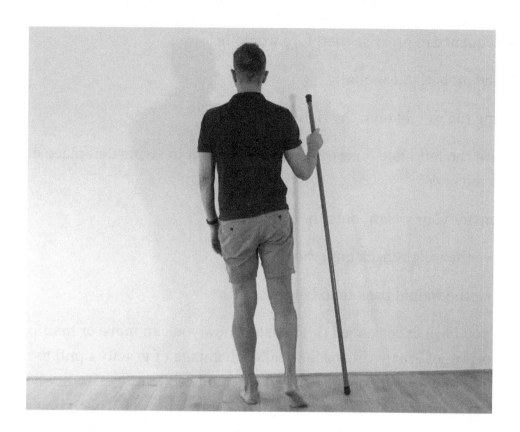

Images 145 to 148: Side and rear view of the transfer of my weight from the right leg onto the left. As I shift my weight, two things happen simultaneously. I begin to reach down with the left side of the pelvis to pour my weight into the left hip, knee, and heel. At the same time I push back with the right leg. Note in the second image from the side that, at the moment the transfer takes effect, my left hip is over the knee and over the heel. In the last image from the rear, you can clearly see from the difference in height of the two buttons at the back of my shorts that I have now arrived on the left leg in our familiar side-bending position. My left side is now longer than my right and I am tall on the left leg.

Pause when you are there, balanced on the left leg, and then bring the weight back onto the right leg, and then back onto your two feet.

Notice that when you bring the weight onto the left leg, it is now the right side of the pelvis that is slightly lifted, and you have this stored up kinetic energy ready to release as you continue forward.

The sequence to practise therefore would be:

1. Stand on both feet equally.

2. Bring the weight onto the right leg.

3. Move the left knee forward allowing the foot to swing and place underneath the knee.

4. Transfer your weight onto the left leg.

5. Move the weight back onto the right leg.

6. Bring the weight back onto both feet.

Once you have experienced this sense of how you can move or manipulate your centre of gravity in space to take advantage of gravity's pull to move forward, you will wonder how you ever managed to move around before. It's a sense of catching the wind in your sails so that you are gliding along rather than falling. Each step is a storing up and a release of kinetic energy around your centre of gravity that uses minimal effort and harnesses the elasticity of your muscles and connective tissue.

Maybe this mental image will help you to sense this.

Imagine that you have a bowl full of water held in both hands. By lowering one hand relative to the other, the weight of the water pours into the lowered side causing the other side to lift, like a seesaw. That enables you to pivot the lighter end forward and then down. As this end lowers outside the base of support, the water (weight) begins to pour into the other end and so on and so forth. The bowl represents your pelvis and the water your centre of gravity. With minimum effort, we are gliding forward and using the physics of gravity to help us as opposed to trying to pick up the tube and its contents and lift it through space, which would be the puppet-like way of moving.

By organising the shape of your centre through side-bending and rotation in relation to the downward pull of gravity you can harness this stored-up kinetic energy to make your walking more efficient, youthful, and graceful.

The key really is to practise. If you have had a hip or knee replacement it will take you some time to learn to trust your new joint, but that is what it is there for so wouldn't it be marvellous to begin to integrate it into your movement?

Once you have explored the sequence in this exercise on both sides, you are ready to take the next step, and then the next, and then the next.

Summary

In this lesson you have learnt how to find stability on the weight-bearing leg and discovered the role that the pelvis can play in the gait cycle. This takes time to develop and there will inevitably be moments when you are going about your daily lives when you will sink back into old habits. It happens to me usually when I am tired and overly focused on something else. I don't get despondent about this, however, but treat it as an opportunity to re-calibrate. I focus on taking a few very mindful steps and I do this by asking myself two simple questions: Am I reaching down into the weight-bearing leg from my pelvis? Am I getting taller? Usually, the answer to at least one of those questions is no, so I slow down, pay attention, and reset.

Enjoy your walking as you build up to longer distances. Walking with your head floating on top of your spine, with your eyes and ears free to scan the horizon, is one of life's pleasures and a great way of staying healthy and independent.

In the next chapter, the second of our focus lessons, we will explore the important skill and challenge of going up and down stairs with confidence.

8 / NEGOTIATING STAIRS WITH CONFIDENCE

Going up and down a flight of stairs is a great opportunity to practise your ability to find stable balance, but for many of my clients who have experienced trauma or joint replacement surgery it's a prospect that fills them with dread.

Here in the UK, many households have their bathroom facilities on the upper floor so not being able to negotiate the stairs with ease can cause huge inconvenience to their daily lives.

The exercises in this chapter will give you the confidence and knowledge you need to overcome your fears and to look upon each journey up and down the stairs as an opportunity to improve your strength, balance, and coordination.

The good news is that, if you have been practising the exercises in the previous chapters, most of what you need to know is already there.

The task ahead is to learn how to apply that embodied knowledge to this functional movement skill in a manner that looks after your joints.

Exercise 24: Bringing the foot up

In the pictures below you will see that I am using a gym step for demonstration purposes along with a stick to help with balance. When I teach this sequence in a group class setting, my students use a portable kitchen step, the kind that can be bought in most larger supermarkets or hardware shops. If you want to practise this at home at the bottom of a flight of steps and hold on to a banister, that, of course, is perfect. Making yourself safe is the important thing and having something to lightly hold on to, whether it be a stick or banister, will help give you a sense of security as you build up your strength and awareness.

The first progression covered in this exercise is to practise bringing your weight onto your weight-bearing leg and placing your free foot onto the step. You have already learnt how to find stability in your standing leg in the previous chapter, so this will seem very familiar.

Stand in front of your step, holding the stick in one hand.

Bring your weight onto your right leg by reaching down with the pelvis to find stability through the hip, knee and foot and think that you are getting taller or longer on the standing leg.

You will find yourself in our very familiar side-bending position. The left side of the pelvis will be slightly elevated compared to the right.

Spend a moment or two here and check that you are breathing and that the jaw is relaxed.

Once you feel stable, lift the left knee, and bring your left foot to rest on the step but do not transfer any weight into it.

Pause for a moment and then bring the left foot back down and come to standing with your weight on both feet again (Images 149 and 150).

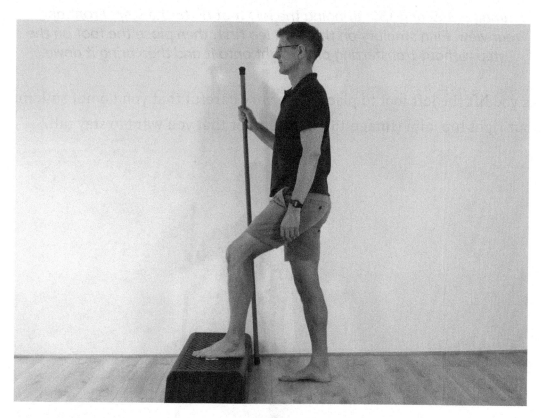

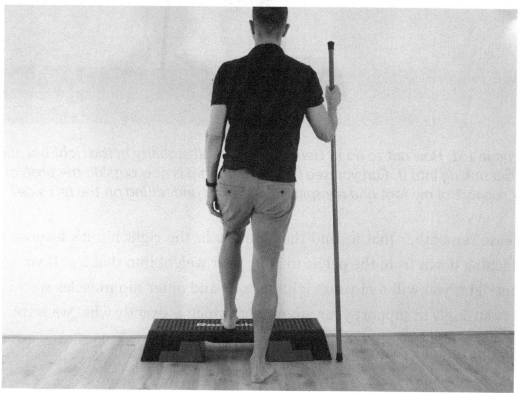

Images 149 and 150: Bringing the left foot on to the step. Front and rear view. Find stability on the right leg first, then place the foot on the step without transferring any weight onto it and then bring it down.

As you lift the left foot to place it, be very careful that you do not sink into your right hip joint (Image 151). Remember that you want to stay tall.

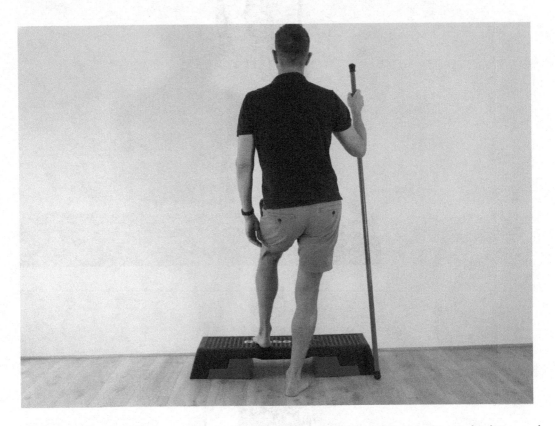

Image 151: How not to do it. Here I have lost all stability in the right hip and am sinking into it. Can you see how my right hip is now outside the base of support of my foot and my spine is distorted and falling on the left side?

Please remember that to find the stability in the right hip it's a sense of reaching down from the pelvis to pour your weight into that leg. If you get this right, you will feel your right buttock and outer hip muscles working very strongly to support your alignment, which is exactly what we want.

Try this on the other side.

Take your time to explore any differences. There's no need to rush. We are working on finding the correct organisation and over time your muscles will adapt.

Pay as much attention to the return of the foot to the ground. It can be very tempting to let go of the stability in your standing leg as you bring the foot down, but the exercise is as much about the coming back as the going up. It's a very deliberate sequence of organised weight transference, and you should be very aware and very deliberate about passing through each stage.

The sequence is:

- The weight is on both feet in standing.
- You shift your weight onto the right leg.
- Bring the left foot onto the step (no weight).
- Bring the left foot back down.
- Transfer the weight from the right leg back to your two feet.

Exercise 25: The exploration of direction

Before we begin the process of transferring weight onto the lifted foot, it will be helpful if you understand the concept of **direction** and how you can use this to help organise your movement.

The concept is best understood by 'doing', which is why this exercise is composed of a series of explorations.

Exercise 25: Exploration 1 The foot-knee-hip connection

Stand facing your step and, as in the previous exercise, bring your weight onto your right leg and place the left foot to rest on the step. This is the start position for the exploration. Keep your weight on the right leg and hip. Your intention is all important here and the instructions are worth repeating because this intention should constantly frame your movement. To keep yourself stable on the right leg you must have a sense of reaching down into the hip, knee, and heel from your centre and lengthening out through the crown of the head.

Pressing into the big toe side

Bring your attention to your left foot and press down a few times into the big toe side of the foot. Press and release. Press and release. Do this slowly and notice what happens to your knee and hip when you press down into the big toe side of the foot (Image 152).

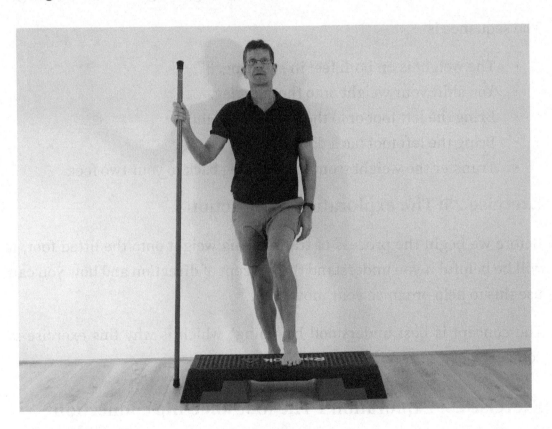

Image 152: Pressing into the big toe side of the left foot. If you look carefully at the picture, you will see that when I press into the big toe side of the foot my knee has shifted inwards towards the midline. This means it is no longer positioned over the centre of my foot. The displacement of the knee has also caused my left hip to move sideways, and I have lost stability in the right hip. This has also caused a twist in the knee. The feet are our foundation, and how we use them has huge implications for how the rest of our movement is organised.

Did you sense how the knee falls to the inside when you bring your weight into the big toe side of the foot and how the left hip displaces?

Once you have explored the effect that relying too heavily on the big toe side of the foot has upon your organisation, it's now the turn of the little toe side.

Pressing into the little toe side

With the same start position, press this time into the little toe side of the foot and notice what happens to the knee and hips (Image 153).

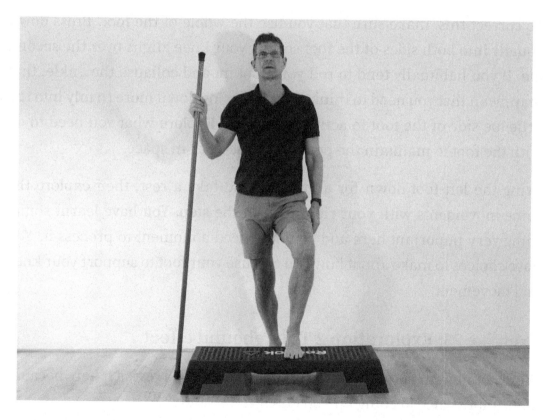

Image 153: Here I am pressing down into the little toe side of the foot to explore what happens to my knee and hips. You can see that my left knee has moved outside the base of support of my foot and my hips have displaced to my right and I am sinking into my right hip. I am once again falling in the sense that gravity has now got a grip on me.

My hope in teaching these explorations is that you will have an embodied understanding of the fact that how you use your foot to bear your weight is important. You will have discovered for yourself that when the weight falls to the inside of the foot, the knee drifts inwards and that when the weight shifts to the outside of the foot then the knee drifts outwards. In neither case is the knee positioned centrally over the foot, and stability is lost in the hips. This means that if you were to then try and stand up on the leg, your weight will not be going through the centre of the knee and foot but will be displaced to one side. It would be a fall rather than a stand.

To correct this, make sure that you use the whole of the foot. Press down equally into both sides of the foot so that your knee aligns over the second toe. If you habitually tend to roll your foot in, and collapse the ankle, that may mean that you need to think about pressing down more firmly into the little toe side of the foot to activate the arch. Explore what you need to do with the foot to maintain the position of the knee in space.

Bring the left foot down for a moment and take a rest, then explore the same movements with your right foot on the step. You have learnt something very important here and you may need a moment to process it. You have choices to make about how you can use your foot to support your knee and movement.

Exercise 25: Exploration 2 The rebound effect

We encountered the 'rebound' effect in Chapter 5 and revisit it here because of its importance to going up and down steps safely.

To begin the exploration, bring your left foot onto the step but keep your weight in the right leg. It is the same start position as in the previous exploration.

Focus on your left foot for a moment and do what you need to do from the previous exploration to align your left knee over the foot.

Then, press down into the foot as if you are pushing the step away from you. You don't need to use a lot of power to do this, but do have the clear intention of pushing down or reaching into the step. Enough pressure to leave an imprint in sand. Press and release. Press and release. Do this slowly enough and at a tempo that allows you to notice what happens to the knee and hip as you press and release (Images 154 and 155).

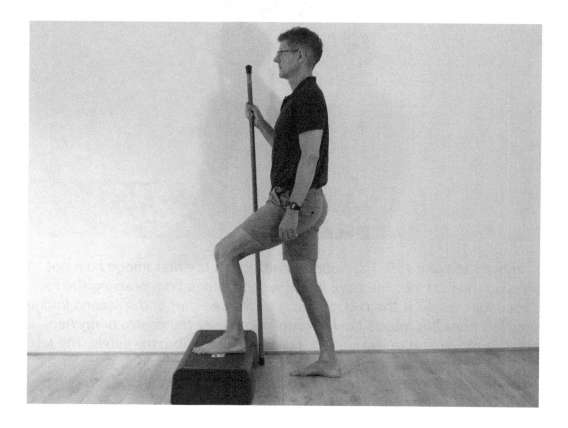

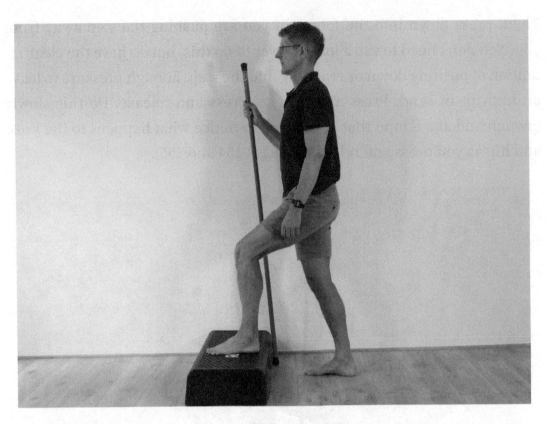

Images 154 and 155: The 'rebound' effect. In the first image I am not pressing the foot into the step; in the second image I am pressing the foot. If you look closely at the two images, you will see that in the second image my left knee has moved back slightly and is over the centre of my heel, and this movement of the knee has created a push into my pelvis. The left side of my pelvis has rotated back slightly. In the first image you can see the outline of my right gluteal muscles; in the second image you can't.

When you press into the foot, the knee 'rebounds' backwards towards the hip. Did you feel that? It's a felt sense of the knee moving towards the knee. As the knee moves backwards it creates a push into the hip socket and you will feel the muscles around this joint begin to engage, ready to bear your weight.

When you stop pressing into the foot, it's a felt sense that the hip is moving towards the knee and the knee is pushed forwards slightly. The knee is in effect falling forward. The hip is falling towards the knee.

The important thing to realise is that if you do not activate the foot and leg by gently pushing or reaching down into the step, you will not be stepping up onto the leg and hip, but you will be falling onto it. It may not feel like a fall, or you may not think of it as a fall because you are not actually going to hit the floor, but it is a fall and to stop that fall you will need to use something else—arm power or other strategies—to prevent that fall.

This is why it is so important that you learn to use the legs and work with this sense of perceived direction to organise your bones so that they are optimally aligned to bear weight and not just put your foot on the step and hope that miraculously things will work out fine. That's a chaotic approach to looking after your health and your movement. You do not want to be falling into the knee every time you go up and down the steps.

It's worth repeating that the direction that you are after is a sense that, as you press into the foot, the knee is moving towards the hip. Not the hip to the knee.

Try this on the other leg before proceeding to the next exercise. The discoveries you will have made in these explorations about how you are currently organising or not organising your movement will be invaluable for the next progression in which we learn how to transfer weight onto the next step. It is time to go up.

Exercise 26: Going up

Stand facing your step. Bring your weight onto the right leg by reaching down into the hip, knee, and heel and lengthening through the crown of the head.

Once you are stable on the right leg, lift your left foot and place it on the step, being careful that you do not sink into the right hip.

Activate the rebound effect by gently pushing the step away from you so that you get the felt sense that the knee is moving towards the hip and not the hip to the knee.

Allow your head to move towards and over the left leg, and as you do this press back and down into the right foot. You will begin to feel a shift of weight through the pelvis as you transition onto the left side. The left side of the pelvis moves back slightly as weight comes into it, and the right side will tilt up and rotate slightly forward towards the left leg. As this happens, allow your head and upper body to continue forwards and over the left leg with the clear intention that the crown of your head is going forward and up (Images 156 to 158).

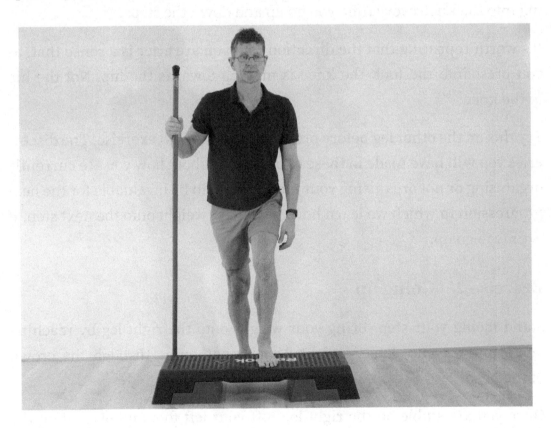

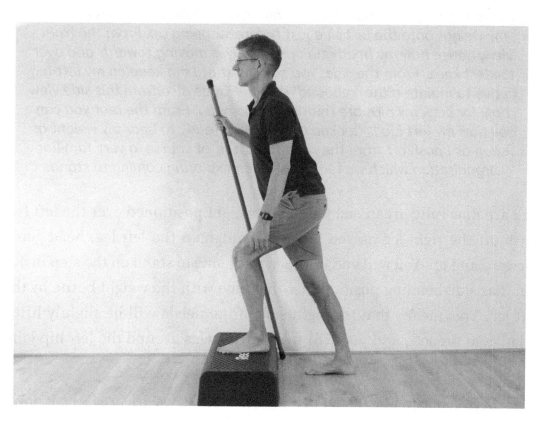

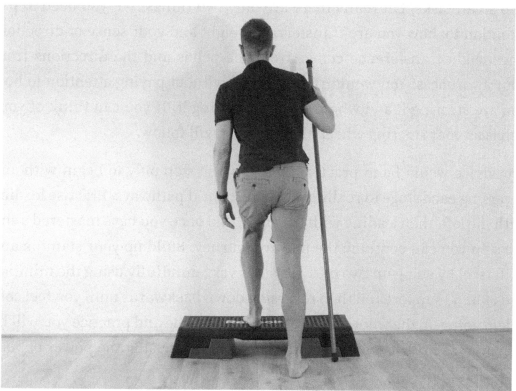

Image 156 to 158: Three views of the moment when I have transitioned my weight onto the left side just before stepping up. From the front view, notice how my head and upper body is moving towards and over the left knee. From the side, you can see that I am keeping my left leg active to maintain the 'rebound' effect. Notice also from this side view how far back my hips are relative to the head. From the rear you can see how my left hip is 'locked and loaded', ready to bear my weight as soon as I push off from the right foot. It is, of course, a very familiar organisation which we looked at when exploring coming to stand.

You are now fully organised with your weight positioned over the left leg. Push off the right leg as you begin to straighten the left leg, head going forward and up. You will end up when you come to stand on the step in our familiar side-bending position, but this time with the weight borne by the left leg. This means that the right side of the pelvis will be slightly lifted relative to the left, and you will feel the muscles around the left hip joint working very strongly to bear your weight.

This may seem complicated to begin with because we are breaking it down into small tasks, but really there are only two things that you need to pay attention to: how you are transferring weight and your sense of direction. The weight transference comes from the pelvis and the directions from your awareness. You wouldn't drive a car without paying attention to how you are steering it and where you are steering it. If you can think of your pelvis as your steering wheel, then the rest will follow.

My advice would be to practise going up one step only to begin with and reversing each stage to really groove the neural pathways. Practise leading with the left, then leading with the right, and once you have mastered a single step you can continue the upward journey. Build up your stamina and skill level by going up two or three steps very mindfully using the minimal use of hand support and then reversing down backwards until you feel confident going up the whole flight of steps. With time and practice you will be able to make the journey up and down the stairs using the power of your legs, hips, and core rather than gripping on for dear life with your arms and trying to pull yourself up.

Going down the stairs

Going downstairs can seem a lot scarier than going up them. This is partly because the downward journey imposes different demands on the way you are lengthening muscles and transferring weight over the non-leading foot.

The following exercise will help you to practise this real-life skill. It's not an easy exercise but one that I have grown, as a teacher, to love. This is because it brings home to a student (myself included), perhaps more than any other exercise, the realisation, and therefore the learning, that the use of the legs does not start at the hip joint but in the pelvis and spine, and that any effective use of the legs is a whole-body event.

Exercise 27: Sideway stepping preparation

Stand sideways on a step with your right side closest to the edge of the step (Image 159).

We will be stepping down with the right leg leading. If you are practising using a flight of steps, then you should practise this at the bottom of the steps, for obvious reasons. A very low step would be a great place to start.

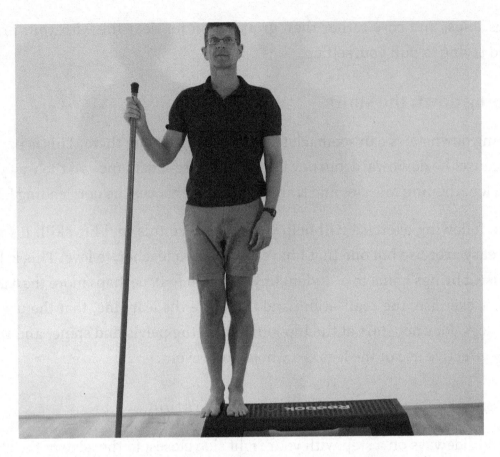

*Image 159: The start position for stepping down to the
side. I am going to step the right foot down.*

Bring your weight onto your left leg in the way that we have explored previously. You will be 'loaded' up onto your left leg in the side-bending position. Your pelvis will be actively reaching down into your left hip, knee, and heel, but you are standing tall. Head is going up. There is no weight on your right leg. The right side of the pelvis will be lifted relative to the left side.

Reach the right foot towards the floor with the leg straight and then bring it back up again. There's no need to go all the way down to the floor to begin with. Practise lowering it a little below the line of the step and then bringing it up again, keeping your weight and head over the left leg (Images 160 to 163). This is difficult so take your time to practise.

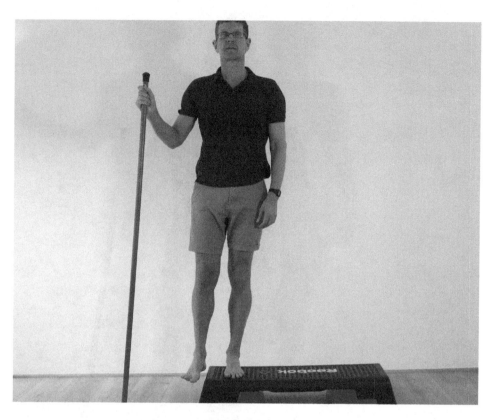

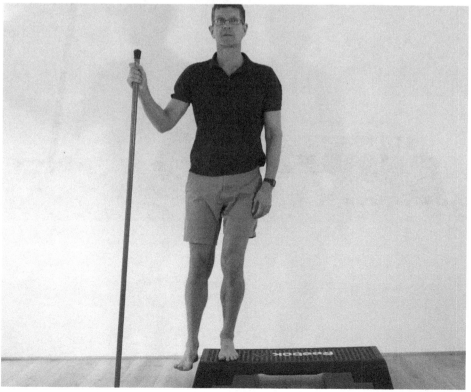

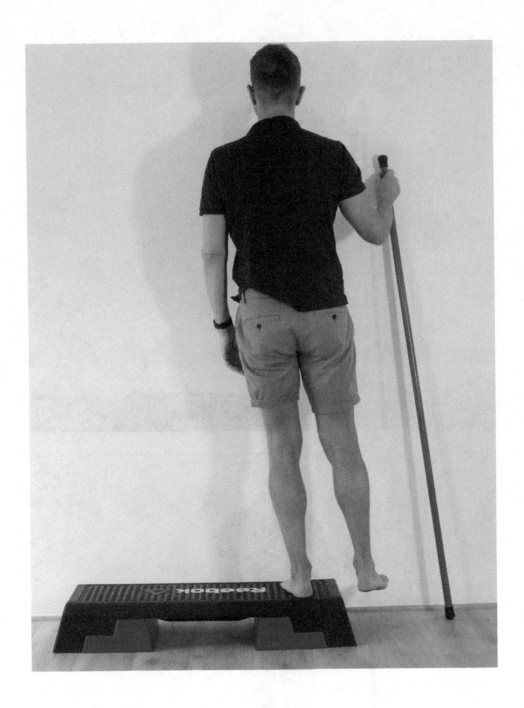

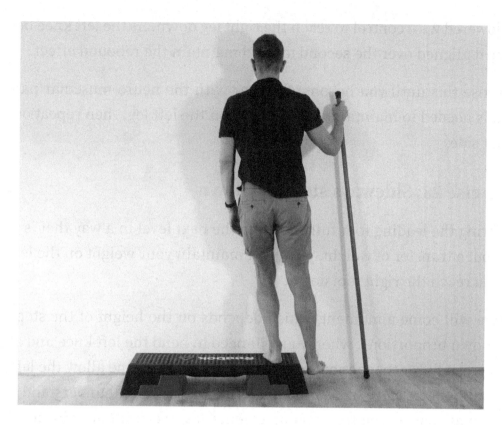

Images 160 to 163: Front and rear views of lowering the right leg from the step. To keep my weight balanced on my left leg and hip as the left knee bends and as the right foot begins to lower, I am working hard on my left side to control the descent. It's a felt sense of actively pulling the left leg actively into me.

To lower the right leg, the sideways curve of the spine has to change. Before you begin to lower the leg, the pattern of side-bending is with the right side shorter than the right, meaning that the curve is over to the left. As the leg begins to lower, it's the left side that has to shorten to control the slow release of the right side. Pay attention to these changes. It will help you if, as you begin to lower the right leg, you actively think of pulling the left leg deeply into your centre. This will help you to keep your balance over the left leg. You will feel the whole of your left side shorten powerfully as the muscles on the left side contract to keep your weight on the left. It is the intensity of this 'grip' on the left side that allows the right side of the pelvis to be lowered with control to reach the right leg down. As the left knee bends, keep it aligned over the second toe and maintain the rebound effect.

Practise this until you become familiar with the neuro-muscular pattern that is needed to maintain your balance on the left leg, then repeat on the other side.

Exercise 28: Sideways stepping down

To bring the leading foot fully down to the next level in a way that is not a fall but a transfer of weight, you must maintain your weight on the left leg as you reach the right foot down.

There will come a moment, which depends on the height of the step and your own proportions, when you will need to bend the left knee and allow it to project over the toes of the foot and at the same time allow the left hip and tailbone to move back as a counterbalance. You will understand what I mean as soon as you try it, but in essence it's a very similar movement to one you have practised before in Chapter 6 when we looked at coming to stand up and sit down with the weight on one leg.

Once the right foot touches down, you allow the weight transference to take place onto the leg. The head shifts up and over onto the right leg which is now your base of support (Images 164 to 166).

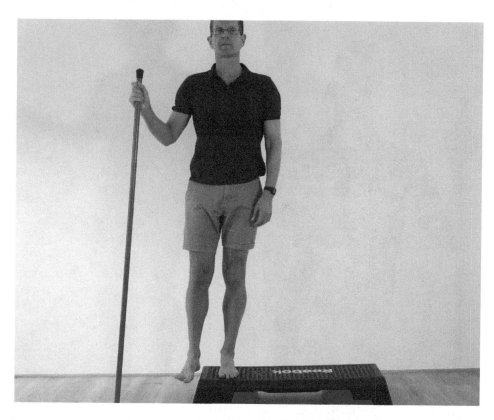

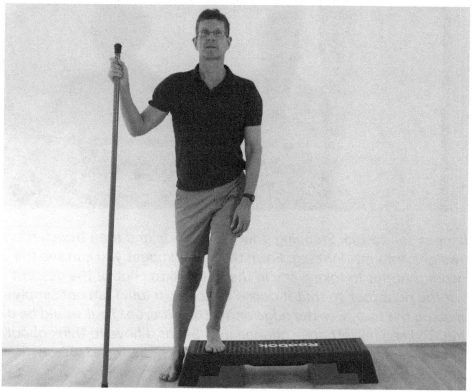

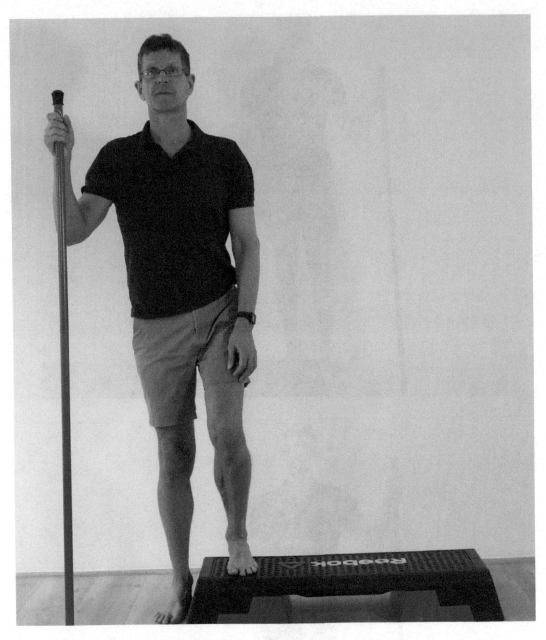

Images 164 to 166: Stepping down to the side and then transferring weight onto my right leg. From the three images you can see the work that has to take place in the left side to control the descent of the right foot so that it doesn't become a fall. I am not simply moving the foot over the edge and letting it drop. That would be a fall. To keep my left knee aligned as it bends, I have to think about how I am using the foot and maintain the rebound effect.

Again, this is something that you should practise until you can do it confidently on both sides.

Exercise 29: Downward stepping progression

The way to progress this exercise is to place the right foot down and slightly forward. You can do this in small increments to begin with until you can place the leading foot in front of you.

This increases the demands on your core to adapt to the movement while keeping your weight on the standing leg. The thing that makes it most challenging is that, as your weight begins to travel forward, your left heel will need to lift as the knee bends. Your weight shifts over the ball of the foot and toes which is a much smaller base of support. This requires a lot of strength and coordination in the ankle and hip. That will take time to establish but, with practice, you will soon be going up and down the stairs with confidence (Images 167 to 169).

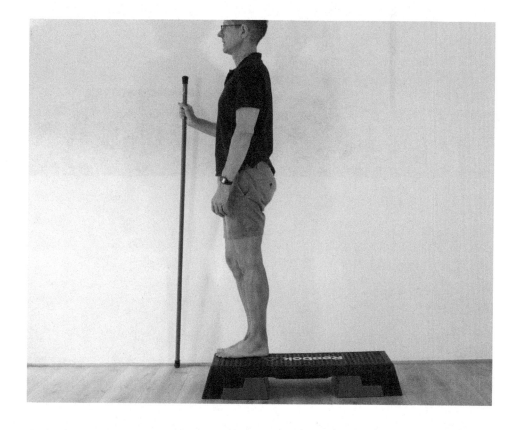

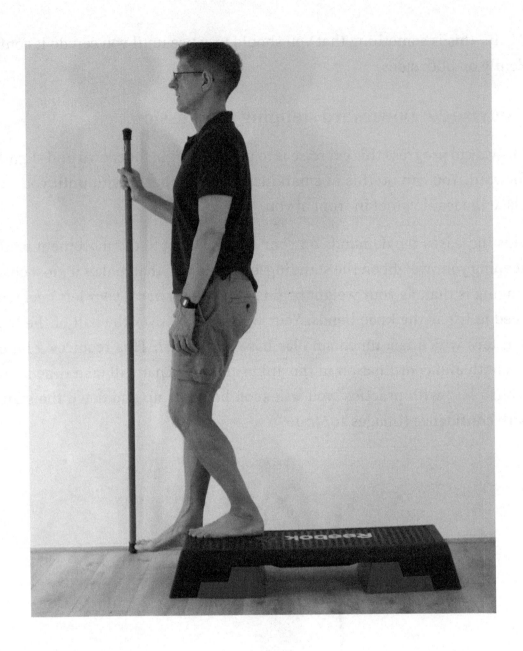

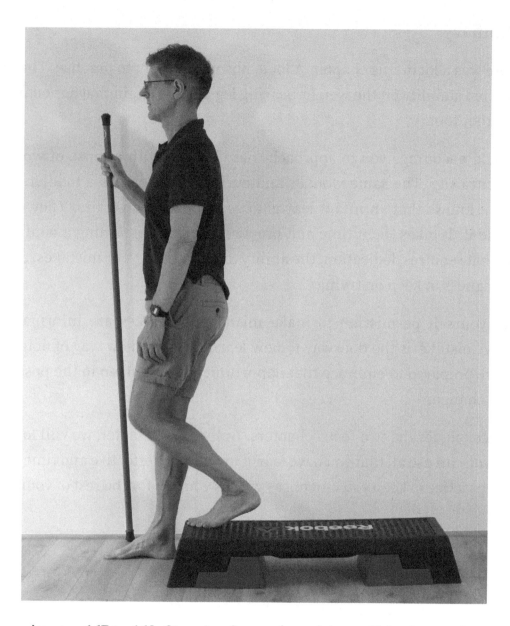

Images 167 to 169: Stepping forwards and down. This places a lot of demand on the weight-bearing leg as the heel lifts and your weight is transitioned onto the ball of the foot and the toes.

Summary

There was a lot in this chapter. A lot to absorb and a lot to practise. The key is to find stability on the weight-bearing leg and maintain that as you place the other foot.

I would encourage you to approach these lessons with a sense of wonder and curiosity. The same wonder and curiosity you had as a toddler. Any parent knows that an infant learns to go up and down stairs. They don't just do it. It takes them time and practice. You are relearning a vital skill and that requires dedication, the ability to learn from your mistakes, and a willingness to keep on trying.

Give yourself permission to make mistakes. Mistakes are information. Every 'mistake' is the doorway to new learning and a new way of doing. If we are prepared to embrace that opportunity, we are open to the possibility of change.

This concludes the two focus chapters. In the final chapter, we will look at how you can use all that you have learnt to create an effective and time-efficient practice to keep you moving as well as you can for the rest of your life.

9 / CONCLUSION

The great advantage of writing a book about the Back for the Future programme is that it has given me the space and opportunity to deep-dive into the 'why' as well as the 'how' of the exercises.

I have always found with my students that if they have a really good understanding of why a movement is helpful for them, then they are much more likely to practise it and to adopt it as part of their day-to-day movement vocabulary.

My mission is not necessarily to get you to exercise more but to move more, and to move more in an intelligent way. As a member of the wonderful Baby Boomer generation, my wish is that you will be able to enjoy the rest of your life to the fullest extent possible, doing all the things you want to do. Nobody wants to be dependent on others as they grow older.

The programme has been designed therefore to teach you how to activate your core and then to teach you how to use your core to initiate intelligent movement.

Intelligent in the sense that your movement aligns with gravity and not against it.

Intelligent in the sense that your movement looks after your joints rather than grinds them down.

Intelligent in the sense that your balance is supported by your core rather than living your life in the state of a constant fall.

This intelligent movement comes when your awareness and your core become a single expression of your intention.

This embodied awareness comes from practice. My practice. Your practice. We are all on this journey together.

At the most immediate level that means, as you begin your journey to better movement, that you make a commitment to practising the exercises and skills outlined in this book on a regular basis, especially if you are what might be called a bit 'stiffer'. You will soon begin to feel the benefits. This is what I call the formal practice.

In my own practice, for example, I will cover the material in the 18 exercises in Chapters 1 to 6, two or three times a week. A session will never take me more than 45 minutes unless I want it to. Sometimes, when time is short and I only have 15 or 20 minutes to spare, I will do fewer repetitions or fewer variations but still shoot through the basic moves: side-bending, long arm reaching, spinal waves, circles, and coming to stand.

I commit to this practice on the chair with the stick because I know it will give my spine a thoroughly good workout in the sense that every direction is explored, and through this practice I am reinforcing my ability to move well in space. I had an accident in my 30s that had a big impact on my ability to move, and that experience taught me that, if I wanted to improve, retain, and keep my mobility, I needed to invest some time and effort into it. I very much wish I had then, the knowledge that I am sharing with you now. It would have made my journey back to health and full mobility a lot easier and quicker.

I never get bored with this material because I take each formal practice as an opportunity to learn something new about the exercises, or the way I am currently moving, and I would encourage you to do the same. The principle I try and follow in my own practice and every class I teach is that no one class should ever be the same. That helps to keep life interesting for me and my students, and you have learnt how to easily introduce variety into your practice.

However, the other way of practising this material, the one that it is really intended to benefit, is real life. The time that you spend away from your chair and stick. All the lessons in this programme have been chosen specifically to give you the skills to improve the way that you move and not for the sake of exercising alone.

I am a huge fan of the work of Katie Bowman, a scientist, movement specialist, and author. If you don't know Katie's work, all her books are well worth a read, but if you only read one then I would heartily recommend her bestselling 'Move Your DNA' (2017: Propriometrics Press).

One of the really important points that Katie makes in her book is that in the West we have tended to fall into the trap of thinking that exercise is movement. We congratulate ourselves on making it to an hour-long yoga or Pilates class, the gym, a swim, a walk, or whatever activity it may be, but we forget that all the other waking hours of the day are an opportunity to bring healthy, nourishing movement into our lives. Even that hour in class, as excellent as it may be, all too often tends to take our joints through limited ranges and habitual movement patterns. That's why Katie is a passionate and eloquent advocate of introducing as much varied movement as possible into our daily lives. I can only and respectfully agree, and it is that shared vision that has inspired me to develop the Back for the Future programme for my clients, many of whom have suffered from a want of such movement in their busy lives and many of whom feel 'excluded' by mainstream exercise protocols.

The skills that you have been learning in the exercises are skills that are directly transferrable into your daily life. That's why they are so useful. The challenge for us all is to take these skills and apply them in our daily life.

Every waking moment is an opportunity for you to initiate movement from your core, provided you are ready to take that opportunity.

Think about how many times you get up and out of a chair each day. Or the number of times you reach for something sitting at a desk or the kitchen table. Or the number of times you go up and down a flight of stairs. Or the number of steps you take in your daily walking.

Even if you consider yourself to be a very sedentary person, it is impossible to negotiate your daily life without movement, and that gives you an opportunity to ask yourself: am I using my core?

Here at my desk, for example, I have a lamp to my right. To turn the lamp on or off I have to reach to touch the switch. I could do that keeping my back rounded, or I could use what I learnt in Chapter 2 to initiate the reach from the pelvis (Image 170).

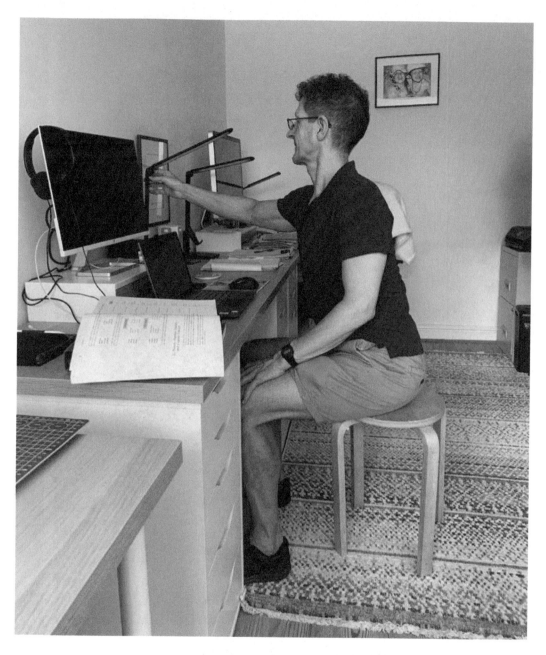

Image 170: Reaching from my core.

To look out of the window I could choose to do that by just moving my neck (I can already feel the strain), or I could use the entire length of my spine to support the use of my head and eyes as we explored in Chapter 3 (Image 171).

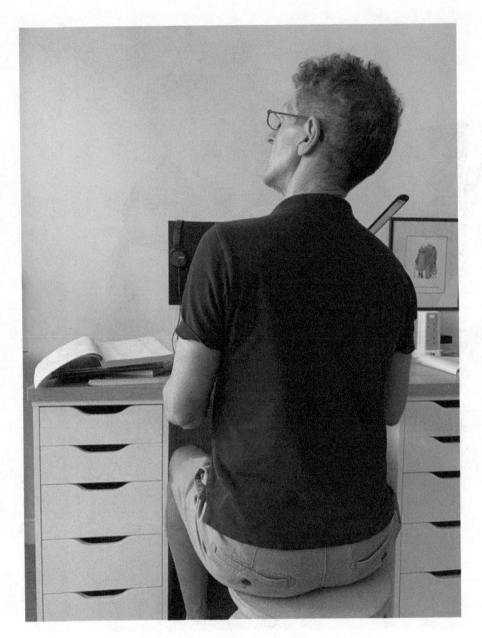

Image 171: Looking out of the window.

To get out of my chair to make a cup of tea, I could push down onto the desk with my arms to stand up, or I could think about how I am transferring my weight into my feet and use the power of my legs to do so (Chapter 6).

To reach for an object on a high shelf I could keep my back rounded and try to lift my arm like a puppet, or I could use this as an opportunity to explore my ability to transfer my weight through side-bending (Chapter 1) onto one leg (Chapter 7) to support the reach of the arm with my spine (Chapters 2 and 3).

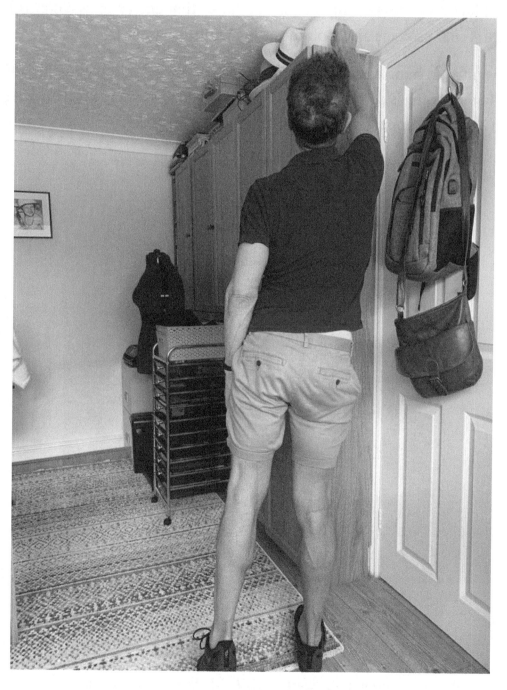

Image 172: Supporting the reach through weight transference, side-bending and extension.

To leave my house I have to walk down a flight of stairs (I live in a coach house). I could do that by tightly holding onto the banister and land heavily on each foot, turning the journey into a series of falls, or I could think about how I am organising my movement so that each step is a controlled descent that protects and looks after my joints (Chapter 8).

If I wanted to hang out the washing, I could do it without paying attention to what my spine is doing, or I could arch my entire spine to keep my weight in my heels to support my vision and arms with my back (Chapters 3 and 7).

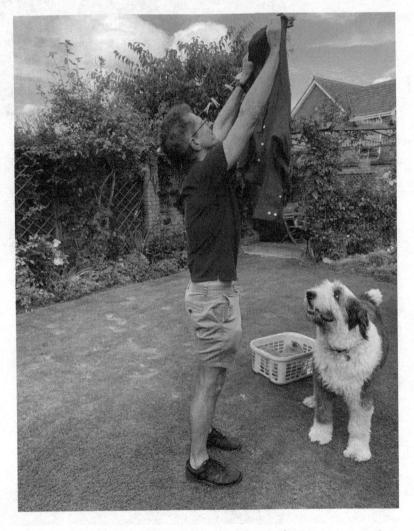

Image 172: Keeping my weight in my heels and using my entire spine to support the reach. Otis, however, had other ideas and wanted me to play!

These are just a few of the examples I could have used.

The point that I am trying to make is that if you want to look after your movement, and transform it for the better, you have so many opportunities to do so. All it requires is a little application on your part to think about how you are moving and a willingness to try your new skills which really aren't new skills at all. It's most likely that you just haven't been using them for a long time. As I said in the introduction, it's not that people can't move in this way. As crazy as it sounds, they have forgotten how. You now have those choices again.

If you want to look after yourself, keep yourself moving, reduce your movement age, stay independent, and feel great then it's time to start moving from your core. This book has given you the knowledge and tools you need to make the choices that support those goals.

Possibly the only person stopping you from doing that is yourself.

I wish you well on that journey to wellness. Please do let me know how you get on. I love to hear from my students.

Stewart

Rutland, UK.

August 2023.

If you have any questions, comments, feedback, or would simply like to share your progress then please contact me via my website: www.stewarthamblin.co.uk.

RESOURCES

My stuff:

For information about my online courses, classes, workshops, and to subscribe to my free newsletter please visit my website: www.stewarthamblin.co.uk

YouTube Channel:

Stewart Hamblin the Feldenkrais Way and Fit Sit®

For more information about the Feldenkrais Method®:

The Feldenkrais Guild UK: www.feldenkrais.co.uk

The Feldenkrais Guild of North America: www.feldenkraisguild.com

Australian Feldenkrais Guild: www.feldenkrais.org.au

For exercise guidelines issued by the UK's National Health Service:

www.nhs.uk/live-well/exercise/exercise-guidelines/

Books:

Alexander, F.M. *The Use of Self.* 1st published 1932. 1985 edition with introduction by Wilfred Barlow. Reissued: London. Orion Books Ltd. 2001

Bowman, Katy. *Move Your DNA: Restore your health through natural movement.* 2nd edition, foreword by Jason Lewis. U.S.A. Propriometrics Press. 2017.

Doidge, Norman. *The Brain that Changes Itself.* U.S.A. Penguin. 2007.

Doidge, Norman. *The Brain's Way of Healing: Stories of Remarkable Recoveries and Discoveries.* U.S.A. Penguin. 2016.

Feldenkrais, Moshe. *Awareness Through Movement: Easy-to-do health exercises to improve your posture, vision, imagination, and personal awareness.* 1st paperback edition. U.S.A. HarperCollins. 1990.

Hanna, Thomas. *Somatics: Reawakening the mind's control of movement, flexibility, and health.* U.S.A. Da Capo Press. 1988.

Kisiel, Jessica. *The Pain Free Athlete: How to Stop Chronic Pain and Achieve Peak Performance.* 2nd edition. Moab, Utah. The Pain Free Athlete LLC. 2018

ABOUT THE AUTHOR

Stewart Hamblin is a UK-based movement specialist, Feldenkrais Practitioner, author of 'The Fit Sit Revolution', and YouTube creator.

For up-to-date information about his classes, workshops, courses, and free newsletter: www.stewarth-amblin.co.uk

YouTube channel: Stewart Hamblin

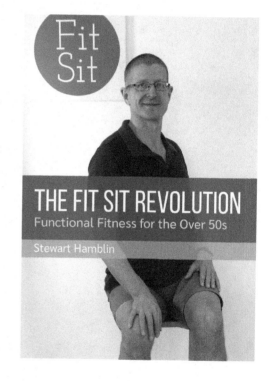

Made in the USA
Monee, IL
16 July 2025

21269215R00157